Breaking Blame

Dr. Schroeder is publishing his first book at age 77.
These are the credentials he offers to his readers:

Distinguished Life Fellow, American Psychiatric Association
Career-long member, American Medical Association
Board Certified in Psychiatry, American Board of Psychiatry and Neurology, 1974
Private practice of general psychiatry, 1973 to 2007
Medical/surgical and psychiatric hospital staff memberships in Orange County, California
Past Clinical Assistant Professor, UCI School of Medicine
Lt. Commander USNR – Camp Pendleton (USMC) Base Psychiatrist, 1971 to 1973
Resident in Psychiatry, UCI, 1968 to 1971
Licensed to practice medicine in California since 1968
Rotating O Internship, Orange County Medical Center, 1967 to 1968
MD degree, Loma Linda University, 1967

BREAKING
BLAME

David Schroeder MD

Published by David Schroeder
Laguna Beach, California
dave@breakingblame.com
www.breakingblame.com

ISBN 978-0-9892085-2-9
Library of Congress Control Number: 2018909459

Book design and illustrations by Jeff Koegel

To Lucile

Contents

Part Two: The World Turned Upside Down

Part Three: When You Know the Notes to Sing, You Can Sing Most Anything

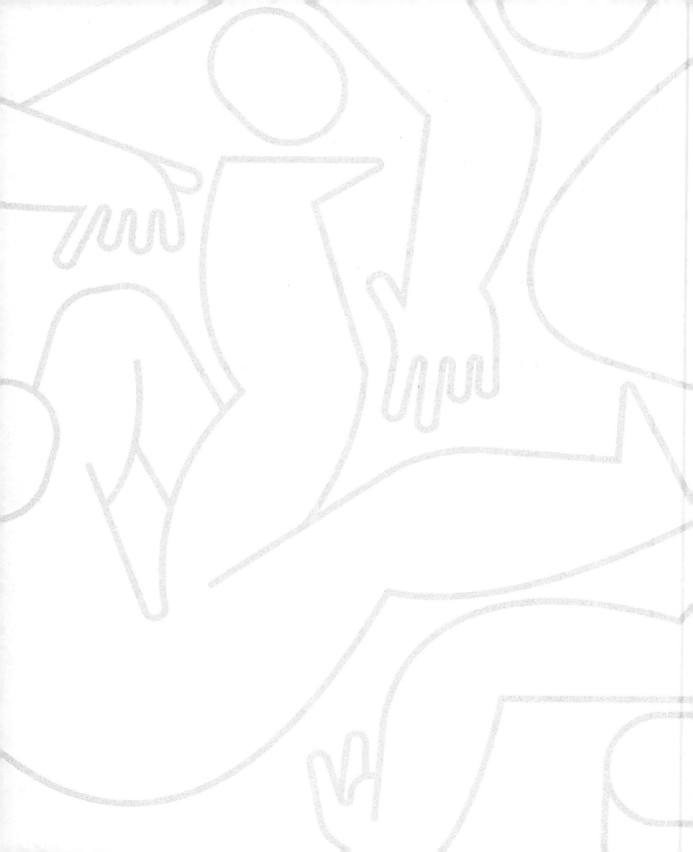

Breaking Blame

If You See Kay

IN 1968 I SURMOUNTED my medical internship at Orange County General Hospital and bagged my California license to practice medicine. I then trooped through three years of training in a psychiatric residency at University of California, Irvine to become a psychiatrist.

The program was brand new; I was the first doctor to complete the entire program. "It was the best of times, it was the worst of times, it was the age of wisdom, it was the age of foolishness, it was the epoch of belief, it was the epoch of incredulity, it was the season of Light, it was the season of Darkness, it was the spring of hope, it was the winter of despair, we had everything before us, we had nothing before us." I'm in awe that Charles Dickens knew 110 years in advance about our educational ordeal, but some of the teachers were horrid, some were OK. Some taught me well the basics of academic, practical, and ethical psychiatry. We had the advantages that came from a fair share of neglect in which knowledge often resulted from deciding what to do, not from learning what to do. The program tried to ace eclecticism, perhaps a euphemism for not knowing what to believe. It was good to be in a place where lofty dogma and doctrine were poorly taught but practicality was consummate. At the time, psychiatric medicines were few in number and less widely used than at present. A major part of those years was spent in the attempt to grasp psychotherapy.

One week out of residency, I was the (singular, one) psychiatrist for the United States Marine Corps Base at Camp Pendleton. I was told that subsumed so many tens of thousands of men that I never believed the number, and I never counted them. We were in the midst of the Vietnam War, so you can imagine I got another practical, figure-it-out-for-myself education. My first instinct was to return a salute by blowing a kiss. Such ignorance of military matters combined with a solid grounding in the practice of medicine made my military tenure the most stress-free and pleasant era of my life up to that point. Quite likely the reason for my ease was the Marines didn't know what to do with a naval officer, the Navy didn't know what to do with a physician, and the docs didn't know what to do with a psychiatrist. I really could—and had to—ad lib as I lived out my onus of the draft.

The day I separated from the Navy, I took off my uniform, insignia, and medal (singular, one) and flung them into the Pacific Ocean; then I went to work in my own private practice in the one office where I remained forever.

I shared rooms and office expenses with Thomas R. Swanson, MD and came to cherish my good fortune of working alongside the man whom I consider to have been the best psychiatrist any doctor could be. We started out as two peas in a pod and ended up thirty-four years later as different as apples and orangutans. We had cleaved into opposite political loyalties, religious beliefs, financial practices, and even sexual orientations, yet I never changed my opinion of him as a doctor, never lost respect or affection for him as a person, and remain ever grateful of my closeness to him.

During the forty years I worked as a doctor, I enjoyed practicing psychotherapy so much it was about all I wanted to do. I didn't have confidence in the methods of psychoanalytic psychotherapy, didn't have the patience for it, and didn't see it as practical. Many of the other techniques such as psychodrama, gestalt, etc. seemed far too theatrical for stodgy me. Hypnosis required a kind of showmanship for which I never had the balls. When cognitive therapy came along, I jumped on it—a chance to actually help patients learn how to think. I have to admit my patience at letting them figure it out for themselves wore short at times, and I would commit the heinous offense of actually telling a patient something.

The common belief ever since Dr. Freud was that patients needed to be studied, seduced, led, beguiled, whatever into discovering on their own the painful, hidden forces and monsters in the subconscious parts of their minds. I was the fool for thinking one should be able to just explain to a patient what was going on. It was believed no one would ever just trust a psychiatrist and learn what the doctor could teach. What worked with shamans, sellers of crystals, motivational speakers, aromatherapists, and purveyors of snake oils would not be accepted from a doctor of medicine? Horrors! One couldn't believe what a professional said unless one first paid for hours and hours of rapport-building sessions and gradually gained insight. Well, I figured if someone were to pay me for sessions, they were already highly motivated to believe what I could teach them, and I would see myself a charlatan if I were to take their money and not send them out of each session with as much teaching as I could possibly cram in.

This is when I started to learn from my patients rather than my teachers. They gave me feedback, intended or not, as to what kinds of interventions were useful, and I began to try with my next patient what had worked with my last. It turns out there are some very important ideas that can be taught and are helpful in increasing both happiness and mental health. One doesn't always have to endure a drawn-out, working-through process. Sometimes what helps can simply be explained and then tried out. In medical school a student sees one (a procedure), does one, teaches one. I found this method can often work with learning happiness as it works with simple surgeries.

Kay is an intelligent woman who had a moderate degree of depression and anxiety when she came to see me in the late 1990s. She is a creative, successful, highly positioned professional who was not going to allow her symptoms to compromise her career or her personal life. She is a quick learner, and her angst decreased rapidly as I taught her what over thirty years of psychiatric practice had taught me about the nature of anxiety and depression. She found my teaching style to be different from what she'd expected based on her previous psychotherapy experiences.

She wanted to know if there were some source in which she could read more of what we discussed. I told her I was just telling it the way I saw it, and I did not know of any written source to which I could refer her. She said, "You've got to write a book." I answered, "I'm not grandiose enough to write a book." She retorted, "You have a moral obligation to write this." We both laughed at her upbraiding as she, by then, knew I didn't believe in morality or obligation. As more years went by, I found about once a week a patient would say to me, "You've got to write a book."

This book is being written at the end of my career, at the end of my life. I was never clever enough to come up with the solutions, pseudo-theories, and philosophies many of my colleagues finessed at the start of their careers. Some of them wrote books early, based only on their training and their own ideas. I had to wait until my patients taught me, and then I took a decade of retirement to mull over what it was they had taught me before I could begin to answer Kay's request.

So, if you see Kay (and in this sentence I use Kay as an exemplar for anyone who would like to become happier and mentally healthier), tell her I wrote her a book—a book which explains the Good News of the joy of being Born Again, this time without the burden of Original Sin.

Introduction

THIS BOOK EXAMINES the concept by which I eventually came to practice psychotherapy. I do not claim my assertions to be facts, but I confidently believe them to be valid. Most important is that accepting them and changing one's behavior in accordance with this concept increases one's happiness and yields a better quality of life for one's fellows. These ideas are also an antidote to the conscious and unconscious thoughts that contribute to anxiety and depression.

My belief is that all normal infants leave toddlerhood with a bogy that they are not good enough until they are better than they are. If they are raised with nothing but praise, there is still the worry that they may not deserve the praise. If they are raised with scolding, they may believe that some fault is theirs. I see the cause of purely psychological anxiety and depression as well as unhappy behaviors as being either reaction formation against such ideas or else direct acceptance of such ideas. No one has 100 percent insight into the existence of such thoughts within themselves, and no one understands completely how such ideas are disguised and embodied in the behaviors that cause unhappiness.

This opinion is not based on faith, nor does it require a knowledge of either esoterica or scholarly tomes. Either I make assumptions and connections which are reasonable to you, dear reader, or you should and will reject them. I also can't claim anything written here to be proven because I haven't thought of any way for a double blind study to confirm or deny what I'm alleging. I easily admit that some patients were not helped by these methods, and I have no data to suggest that my techniques are better than any others. The book is filled with anecdotes, which are not offered as proof of anything. They are used to demonstrate a technique, not as evidence that the technique is better than any other technique.

I believe these ideas are neutral to faith or absence of faith. My patients included Protestant ministers, Catholic priests, Jewish rabbis, Buddhists, agnostics, and atheists. I have discussed these ideas with evangelicals and anarchists. I have yet to change or try to change the faith, or lack of faith, of anyone. More important: I've never met anyone who found my ideas to disagree with their beliefs once we talked long enough to understand the implications of both their beliefs and my concept. This will be elucidated in chapter 6.

I have the same belief that everything I have written is consistent with ethical, traditional, and academic standards for the practice of medicine and psychiatry and is at no variance with current teachings of accredited medical schools and the American Medical Association and the American Psychiatric Association.

Wherever I've made reference to one with whom I've had a confidential contact, both the names and the circumstances have been altered to ensure privacy, but the psychological nature of the stories is true. The names used in non-confidential relationships are actual, and the circumstances and events of the stories are undisguised.

I give credit to Anne Curzon, PhD, who through her lectures for the Great Courses, moved me to adopt the singular *they* as my third person pronoun of choice when referring to one whose gender is not in evidence.

For one to advance beyond one's present capacity for happiness, it is not enough to learn

new material to add to what has already been learned. One must go back and re-examine the central

ideas of what was believed originally and make changes to those core beliefs

— then learned by the mind of an infant —   *on the basis of what today is adult wisdom.*

PART ONE

You Must Be Born Again

1

Gripping the Racket

IN COLLEGE I WAS LUCKY to have friends who were more athletic than I. A few of them took me under their wings and taught me to play tennis. I loved the game and worked at improving my skills for a couple of decades until I thought I was up to mediocre. After I'd been in medical practice for a forever or two, I decided to buy lessons from a professional to learn to play better than what I had thought was so-so.

I expected a teacher would start with me at my current level of play, and I'd progress from there. Duh! I wasn't holding the racket correctly. I didn't know how to place my feet. My first motion to move the racket was all wrong. As I progressed, I found no matter how much I improved, my tennis pro was just as enthusiastic in pointing out microscopic errors in the tiniest details such as a wrist angle resulting in misplacement of the face of the racket.

Using all that my friends had taught me in college and working hard for years to improve had left me with the firm belief that I had little aptitude for athletics and would have to work very hard to be a less than average tennis player. Erasing what they had taught me and starting over with a new grip, new stance, and new way of moving my body showed me my lack of natural ability was far less a handicap at playing than I had thought.

Happiness is like tennis. If you're going to learn to be happier, you have to go back and start at the beginning and do a different beginning. Misconceptions and falsehoods were taught to you for decades, and you have based your behavior and beliefs on those errors. If those errors are corrected, you will find that being happier than you had thought possible will be analogous to my becoming a more skilled tennis player than I had thought possible.

During the years my tennis pro was correcting my nuances, I happened upon a young stud teaching his girlfriend to play tennis at a local park. He repeatedly tossed the ball over the net and yelled, "Hit it." He added multiple encouragements and assurances peppered so liberally with "Fuck, YES" or "You can fucking do this" or "You're just fucking great" that I began to suspect he either had a limited vocabulary or had attended a Tony Robbins Date with Destiny. This was not a tennis lesson. He didn't have the expertise of my instructor, and the only thing he was doing for his friend was enticing her into believing in herself. The world doesn't need another self-help book that provides hype, encouragement, orgasmic glee, or the negation of any supposed sins—no matter how much it may be peppered with either fucks or praise Gods. You can't change your permanent level of happiness by listening to those who inspire. Telling those who are unhappy or depressed to love themselves is like telling a novice pitcher to throw strikes.

My tennis master was a model for my idea of therapy. He taught truer basics as a replacement for what had been provided by my college friends. Then he built on the corrected basics as he showed me how to play. The guy in the park was a model for the self-help purveyors of drivel who write books and make big bucks emitting encouragements and saying nothing more than "Don't worry, be happy." Uplifting rhetoric will draw in both crowds and profit, and the guy in the park may have been more successful at getting laid than my tennis club pro, but one cannot learn to be a tennis player from him, and one cannot learn to be happier from those touting positive platitudes.

In this nascency one must learn that there is no better. Worse and better, good and bad, right and wrong, and guilt and innocence are false concepts and have no place in the emotional structure of a happy adult. Punishment is never appropriate. These are deceptions, ubiquitous deceptions to be sure. Throughout the rest of this book, I will explain what I mean and teach how to apply it in life. My goal is not to pose a philosophical argument. It is to increase happiness and well-being.

A word about my insistence in going back to the beginning: I do not mean having the patient talk about their beginning. I intend that the therapist teaches the patient what the patient couldn't learn as an infant but now needs as basics. The experience with my tennis pro did not involve me telling him what had happened to me with my college mates or earlier, and it did not require me to expose my past athletic embarrassments. He didn't need to hear my grief at having been the last one chosen whenever my grade school chums would be forming teams at recess. I simply needed to be willing to let him teach me the beginning steps as new. Patients often told me about earliest memories, and the telling would provide meaningful examples to bolster what I was teaching, but I did not ask them to tell me early memories or to go back and excavate the buried treasures or detritus in their minds.

With some common techniques of psychotherapy, the patient dredges up the early traumas involved in the development of their neuroses. It's as if there are monsters cached in the closets and under the beds of their psyches. Each dark space is probed for the monster to be extracted and shown to be not a monster at all, only a misunderstanding. I believe the rapping on the wall outside a patient's consciousness does not always call for a scary journey into the cold night to discover that it is a tree branch and not a monster banging on the mind. My conviction is patients can be taught in the present that there are no monsters, and their behavior and thinking can be coached into harmony with a happier life not warped by infant fantasies, just like my tennis pro could teach me the basics and then coach me on how to use those basics to begin playing more skillfully.

When a patient would learn the absurdity of monsters, they would more easily bring up the memories of their childhoods that had engendered the traumas, but these then would be anecdotes to illustrate and encourage growth, not heartaches.

What I am referring to as a monster is any belief that the patients, or you, were ever wrong, blamable, guilty, bad, or deserving of shame.

My sports analogy fails in one specific, a failure I want to air because I think it could mislead. My having learned basic errors in tennis happened because my instructing buddies didn't know any better how to teach, but having learned basic errors in early childhood did not occur just because the teachers didn't know better; it was because an infant doesn't learn with the mind of a college student. The mind of an infant is a maelstrom of misconstruction—and, too, their teachers didn't know any better.

One who wants to learn the basics of being happier has a real problem finding teachers who are experts in the necessary nuances. I'm hoping this book can relate my concept of what it is that needs to be taught, but I humbly admit that no manual is as effective as a teacher. I will be describing what is my style of psychotherapy because it helped Kay; it's what I developed in my practice, but I can't claim it to be any better than what is done by a multitude of expert psycho-therapists. Those data don't exist.

Ignorant do-gooders, on the other hand, we have with us always. Every Tony, Rick, and Werner claim to be—and have an army of groupies endorsing their claims—purveyors of exper-tise and guidance. A friend introduced me to a new age traveler recently, telling her that I was a psychiatrist. Her response to me was, "Oh, we're colleagues; I'm an aromatherapist." A young acquaintance with a stunning torso who works as a personal trainer at my local gym told me he doesn't need college; he plans to make a career of sharing his happiness. I suspect he could spread more happiness sharing his body than his mind, but—alas—that's not what he intends.

No matter how real is the problem of knowing which teachers to trust, one has to either invent the entire universe for oneself or else be taught. Choose your teachers the best you can, and be ready to move on to others if new understanding dictates. Remember, science observes and admits it doesn't know but is trying to find out. Belief says it does know and refuses to risk being misled or confused by emerging data. For me, observation trumps belief.

"The problem with the world is that
the intelligent people are full of doubts,
while the stupid ones are full of confidence."

CHARLES BUKOWSKI

Original Sin

WHEN EXPERIENCING YOUR FIRST GO at life, you had the mind of a neonate, an infant, a toddler, then a preschooler. By the time you got to kindergarten, your personality and your perception of reality, just like your first verbal language, were pretty much formed–formed in a mind that had next to nothing in the way of knowledge, wisdom, judgment, information, experience, and abstract reasoning. I'm using the idea of being Born Again to describe the fantasied accomplishment of going back to the cradle and beginning anew to develop a self-perception based on the best reality, wisdom, judgment, information, experience, and abstract reasoning available to an adult mind. You couldn't do that the first time through! A baby can never have an adroit mind at its disposal while it is forming its perceptions. As adults, the core of our knowledge about ourselves and our milieu is based on an infant's misperceptions of what they were sensing. And that infant was then taught by those who didn't know what they themselves were about.

I assign the term Original Sin to that very first tort done to all infants when they are wrongly taught to accept themselves only conditionally. In those first years, they are insidiously brainwashed—convinced that they are either bad or good. No infant has in them—or has ever been—good or bad, but their misperceptions of the world will convince them that such is the case before they leave toddlerhood. This faulty acceptance becomes the concrete foundation upon which the brick-and-mortar prisons and torture chambers of anxiety, depression, and unhappiness are erected in later stages of life.

Even more damaging than how we are taught to think is how our physical bodies are conditioned to respond. Pavlov rang a bell before feeding a dog. He noticed after a while the dog would get biologically ready for food not from seeing or smelling food but from hearing the bell. The bell alone, without any food being present, would cause the dog to salivate and secrete stomach acid.

In Pavlov's dog the bell had been paired with food resulting in the bell causing those bodily changes that previously the food had caused. In the infant anything unideal is paired with scolding resulting in anything less than perfect causing biological changes of angst. Hang on to your objections about my use of the idea that all infants are scolded. I don't mean it as it sounds and will explain anon.

I'm alleging that ten-thousand times before a child completes toddlerhood someone will scold them when something untoward is experienced by the child, thus the child will enter a biological—as well as psychological—state of dysphoria whenever anything happens not to the liking of the child. I don't know if this takes more time or less time than it took Pavlov to condition his dog, but it does happen well before a kid is out of the high chair.

I used the word scold in the above two paragraphs in a sense so wide that an explanation is needed. I mean the word to include any sense of abasement or discouragement, even though such was never intended by the caretaker. This includes most of the early attempts to comfort in that comforting can be perceived by a developing mind as a message that it should not be upset. If something makes the child sad and the comforter tells the child, "Don't be sad," then—in the strange sense with which I'm making this statement—the child is being discouraged (scolded) for being sad even though the message is meant to be consoling and is said in a most loving coo. In coming up with my ten-thousand event estimate, I'm including all the comforting, consoling, condemning, and confusing messages that accompany all untoward perceptions on the part of the infant, toddler, and child.

The above paragraph seems silly to me if I misunderstand it like some ignorant who hears about the theory of evolution and then scoffs at the idea that a monkey turned into him and goes on to grunt that if this were so why do we still have monkeys. Obviously, there is no single age in the development of a person that the above happens, just like it didn't happen that an ape became a man. But if one were to summate the experiences of an infant, a toddler, and a preschooler and realize that society does the same thing to each person as it becomes an adult, one can see that innumerable conflicts arise over any emotion associated with an angering or saddening occurrence. Even adults do not know how to be sad or angry without marrying that emotion to some sense of failure, weakness, guilt, or blame, even if it is so simple as to feel that they shouldn't be as sad or angry as they are.

For any given infant, I believe there are biological responses to any perceived negativity. If an infant is hungry, cold, deprived of sleep, or in pain, something changes in the chemical and the neurological function of the infant. It's far beyond my learning or the scope of this book to pursue what psychophysiologists have learned about all this. I just need to make, and therefore use, the point that these things do happen.

It is probably a good thing lie-detector results are not accepted in court. The results are at too much risk of misinterpretation, since the responses of no two persons are the same. But no one disputes that telling a lie can cause changes in blood pressure, pulse, respiration, and sweating that can be picked up by the polygraph. I think all would also accept that a person prone to severe blushing secretes blood vessel dilating hormones when they are embarrassed. The cause for ulcers has been found to be far more complicated than thought when I was in medical school, but no one denies that emotional distress can cause stomach pain—just as it's widely accepted that stress can cause heart attacks.

Some persons seem resistant to these kinds of biological changes brought on by subtle emotions, but others are highly susceptible. There are those who will blush at such minimal stress that one never figures out why. When such a person fears they are blushing, they may blush more. If you point out the blushing, that may trigger a far more profound vasodilation. I have had my leg quaver uncontrollably just because of the onset of sexual excitement or fear, and clearly one's blood chemistry is different if one is proud than if one is ashamed.

To summarize and reinforce in the minds of my readers, I am averring that the result of Original Sin is merely (!) that a developing human is conditioned, from infancy and until death, to respond physically (brain chemistry, neurology) and psychologically (emotions) and enter a state of shame, blame, guilt, or angst any time anything is not as desired. A purpose of this book is to teach how to experience sadness and anger absent the sense of anxiety or depression.

When I was in my early forties, my parents and I were having a fun chat about the old days, and I told them my earliest memory was of me standing in the driveway of the house we lived in when I was born, looking at a window, and feeling overwhelming, catastrophic shame as if I had ruined the world. I can still remember that horrid wanting to not exist. My parents were shocked, and both agreed in all details of what they then told me. During World War II, they had rented a room to a young woman whose husband was away in the fight. She had put a radio in her bedroom window and had draped the antenna wires down the side of the house at the driveway. I had been playing alone in the drive and tugged on the wires. The woman came out of the house, scolded me, and spanked me. I have no memory that woman ever existed. I don't remember the scolding or the spanking. This punishment, I was told four decades later, started a row—which I'm told I witnessed—between my mother and the tenant. My world (at that age I was aware of nothing outside of my home) was at war because of something I had done absent any motive on my part to either offend, cause trouble, or disobey anything. The resultant conflict between the war bride and my mother convinced me I wasn't good enough for this world, and the result was, to me, cataclysmic. The only thing I had remembered was some vague sense of me outside that window, devastated beyond comprehension because some unknown inadequacy in me was destroying my universe. The thing about my memory that most shocked my parents was they recalled moving from that house when I was twenty-three months old, and neither of them could recall how long before we moved this event had occurred. I suspect they may have been one year off in their calculation.

I was recently using this story in a chat with my adult children to illustrate that the malignancy of Original Sin is that it causes us to be unable to experience pain, sadness, grief, or anger without evoking shame or guilt just like Pavlov's bell evoked the saliva. David Jr. reminded me of an event that occurred when he was about four years old which reinforces even better my thesis that anything unpleasant will cause shame or guilt or blame. On the afternoon my wife and I took our three children to see a weekend matinée of *Mary Poppins,* David fell and broke his arm at the restaurant where we had stopped for lunch on the way to the cinema. Instead of seeing the movie, we spent the afternoon in an emergency room. As an adult, David said he remembered nothing of the pain of breaking the bones or of having them set. He remembered his guilt at depriving his siblings of seeing the movie.

My tennis-playing college friends didn't know what was known by the athletic professionals who taught me later in life, so they couldn't have taught me any better than they did. Your parents, mine, and Drs. Freud and Phil didn't know and weren't able to teach us how to start out life either. Even if they had, one can't teach reality to an infant mind any more than one could coax a backhand swing from a crawler. So likewise, the brainwashing, which I am calling for lack of a better idea Original Sin, could not have been prevented no matter how wise the parent. But here's hope: as adults it can be made obvious to us if we want a better backhand, want to speak a foreign language, or want to master a musical instrument, we will have to learn something new. We also need to learn something new—and it has to replace what we wrongly learned before—if we want to be happier, more mentally healthy adults. Just as I could never be a skilled tennis player until I gave up my unfortunate grip and swing, likewise we can never be happier until we give up our unfortunate concepts of good/bad, right/wrong, and shame/guilt—all of which are nothing more than the result of Original Sin.

In late toddlerhood, children are encouraged to give up the infantile disinterest in bowel and bladder control. At grade school age, they are supported in giving up beliefs in Santa Claus and the Tooth Fairy, but no one ever teaches them that some of the most basic concepts that cause their later proneness to depression and anxiety are even more infantile and false than their beliefs in sprites and fat men who can visit hundreds of millions of homes on the stroke of midnight. Relatives, co-workers, lovers, law enforcement, the law courts, teachers, doctors, clergy, and even our own children constantly, but erroneously, reinforce the false ideas that good and bad, blame and shame, and right and wrong are real.

I don't think one can ever get all of the effects of right/wrong thinking out of one's head, but one can learn to get rid of much of it, and the more one drops it the greater is one's potential for happiness and mental health. Hanging on to the infantile idea of right/wrong when grown up actually does cause more dysfunction than if one were to go through adulthood pissing and shitting one's pants and believing in Santa Claus and the Tooth Fairy.

I am aware that I have not yet discussed how or why concepts of good and bad are false and only the result of Original Sin. I renew my promise to field this discussion soon (chapter 6), but for now I'm only attempting to make the point that this misfortune did happen to you like everyone else, and it has eclipsed your potential for happiness. (I was discussing this concept with my friend Laura [of whom you'll soon read more] when she confronted me with the confusion caused by my use of Original Sin when I don't believe in sin. She suggested that I just call it what it is—Bullshit. Yes, Laura, I don't believe in sin, but I do believe in manure. So for the rest of the book, it's just going to be called BS.)

3

The Omnipotent Infant

WHEN YOU WERE NEW, you were aware of no one other than yourself and, later, your primary caretaker. That was your universe. When you cried, the entire universe responded to your cries. You soon learned you could get that universe to smile, frown, feed, warm, and clean you—the omnipotent who could summon the gods and the devils. Nobody told you there were billions of people in the world who all think and act differently from each other. Even more, the infant is aware of no activities of the caretakers other than caring for the baby. Every being in existence only takes care of you; they are of no purpose, whatsoever, other than tending to you. What they did say, you saw as coming from the universe, Truth. If they said you were good, then you were good. When they said you were bad, then bad you were.

Adults usually see this as a period of helplessness for an infant because of all the things the infant cannot do, but the infant is aware of none of the functions they lack. The infant knows no existence save that of which they are the center. They are aware of no power other than the power they have. The infant grows into and out of these perceptions, of course, which aren't the same during different weeks of the infant's life, but this conceit on the part of the infant is a misperception of reality that gels, much of which life doesn't notice to correct.

For obvious reasons, good and bad got instilled in those first years, and—for equally obvious reasons—consequences and responsibility were nonexistent concepts until a later state of development. It is, therefore, no surprise that our adult concerns over whether we are bad or good are actually more central, more primordial than our worry over consequences. A most trivial example would be that often an adult will break something and feel worse about their having broken it than they do about it being broken. Non-trivial examples would be patients coming to me with depression caused by guilt over something they had done long after the consequences of the action had become irrelevant. "Don't cry over spilled milk" is only a cliché because people cry over the fact they spilled the milk, even longer than over the milk being wasted.

As a toddler, when I toddled into the street, I wasn't told about the dangers of colliding forces. I was somehow made to feel I was bad—or I had done something bad. OK, so there are enlightened ones now who won't use the word "bad." Sorry, enlightened ones, a frown, a prohibition, or a nudging the infant away from a danger are all equally interpreted by that omnipotent infant as bad. And remember, it isn't the caretaker who is telling the infant they are bad at that instant—it is the whole universe.

Somehow, in the most liberal or in the most puritanical environment, the infant learns staying on the lawn is right but running into the street is wrong. Doing "it" in the toilet someday becomes cool, but finger painting the walls with shit is somehow UGH. Again, those words to the infant are all the same as good/bad, right/wrong, sin/righteousness, and safe/dangerous. The kid can't abstract the nuances.

Colby, a man in his fifties who was successful in marriage and business while at the same time a very athletic surfer dude, became a patient of mine because he was having anxiety attacks. Outwardly he had all the trappings of a worry-free life. He was wealthy, healthy, and wise. He did well in therapy and learned to handle his biological symptoms with insight, which relieved psychological components as well. During a session late in his treatment and at the end of a calendar year, Colby told me that during the previous week a long-forgotten memory surfaced from his days in the small New England town where he had been raised until age five.

He had been in a nativity play at his nursery school on Christmas Eve. Later that night he had begged to open one Christmas present, but the request had been denied. The next day he had been excited to rip into his presents but again had to wait. He had not been allowed to open any package until weeks later. His parents had been annoyed with him as he kept up the begging, and he had interpreted their crossness as evidence of his unworthiness to ever get any presents. He, mister captain of macho (said with all respect, not sarcasm), burst into tears as he related to me that when the memory surfaced a few days prior to our session, he pictured himself in big, black boots and a clumsy, worthy-of-wonder hat in that pageant. It only now, as an adult, dawned on Colby that his costume had been that of a pilgrim in a Thanksgiving vignette. I remember his sobbing summation: "All those years I thought I was such a bad boy I didn't deserve any presents, but I was just confused about which holiday had been celebrated that night." The only awareness of his loving and generous parents had been that he was excited about Christmas and impatient. I suspect that it might (or not) be significant that the memory never surfaced during his adult years until he learned to be unafraid of his anxiety.

Notice, there is no suggestion that Colby's parents had done anything to instill in him the notion he wasn't good enough. It had been his perception, of which his parents were unaware, that if he weren't able to open his gifts the cause had to be himself—that he was bad. By that age it could have been explained to him if anyone had understood his misperception. He was old enough to understand days and calendars, but the fallback position was a remnant of infantile omnipotence.

A devastating and universal materialization of infantile omnipotence fused with BS is suffered by children of divorce. At the right age (which differs for each child) comes the surety that they are to blame for what to them is a catastrophe. The connections they make are astounding. My great-nephew thought he was responsible for his parents' separation because he had voiced unhappiness with his school.

At an early enough age, a child can't understand or verbalize their own feelings and certainly can't sort out the feelings coming from their caretakers. The most loving attempt at comfort from a kind parent might be perceived in some way as similar to a rebuke from a harsh parent. At puppy training school, I learned the corrective effect on my dog of the pronunciation of a sharp "Eh!" Let's be in wonder about the effect on a toddler of hearing an "Oops!"

I don't want to hold forth with a psychiatric discussion—such as I was subjected to during my post-internship residency in this medical specialty—of every possible misconception. I can't claim to know what goes on in New Guinea, Samoa, Bhutan, or Madagascar, but any child raised in Western society is affected by this kind of conditioning thousands of times before they reach an age which they will be able to remember. An adult will revert to such omnipotence when they come across a mean person and wonder what they did to cause them to act that way.

So here we are as adults arguing politically, legally, religiously, and philosophically (and effecting happiness and mental health) over concepts of morality, ethics, goodness, and what all else based on the infantile belief that there is right and wrong, good and bad—a fiction. Consequence and responsibility are almost irrelevant in the thinking we do without thinking about our thinking compared to those primitive ideas of good and bad. In our culture, still when we are adults, doing something with sad consequences is less a cause for concern than doing something bad. If I hurt you, I will care that you were hurt, but I may worry more about whether or not I was bad—or how bad I was—to have done so. This morning I bumped heads with my teenage granddaughter, with me getting a major bruising. Darla was so sorry she had bumped me first, checking to see if I was OK second.

"The universe is under no obligation
to make sense to you."

NEIL DEGRASSE TYSON

4

Saved from the BS by the SOB

ABOUT THE TIME INFANTS BECOME children, a balance—a scale of justice—develops in them that gives them an out from the BS. If anything is not as desired, a Shift of Blame (SOB) allows for the absence of shame if it is the other guy's fault. This exception to the omnipresent I'm-not-good-enough belief becomes a second option whenever something is amiss. Picture yourself on a teeter-totter. If I'm down, you're up. I can't be up unless you're down. Please, just replace the words up and down with shame and blame. If there's an imbalance in life, it's to your blame or else it's my shame.

I want candy. I don't have candy. Mommy gives me candy. I'm happy I got candy. So far so good. Or, I want candy. I don't have candy. Mommy does not give me candy. I'm mad I did not get candy. So far so good. I'm happy if I get what I want; I'm mad if I don't get what I want. Next comes the BS. I should not be mad I don't have candy, because candy is not good for me, or there's something (bad) about me that prevents me from having candy. Then I may stay dysphoric—I'm not what I should be. I'm wrong to be angry, or I'm not good enough to have candy. The other option is that I am fine to be what I am (angry) because Mommy is mean. It's me or it's her, but one of us is to blame for me being angry about not having candy. If I'm not angry, there is no problem. But if I didn't get any candy, I am angry, and it's my fault unless there is a Shift of Blame to it being her fault.

One childish, malignant step more: if I am hurt by some experience, I will tend to feel some degree of shame unless I can blame another. If the other is to blame, I will experience some degree of shameful helplessness unless I can see the other punished. In making this statement I am telescoping many stages of psychological development. Just to make it easy to remember, I oversimplify it into the idea that when something ill occurs, a toddler will feel shame, a child will blame, an adolescent will defame (the girlfriend who dumped me is a slut), and an adult will retain (an attorney to sue the crap out of you).

I'm claiming it to be universal because it surfaced in those experiences which really are universal—or at least culture wide. We all pooped places they didn't want us to poop. We all wanted more than we got. We all suffered pain that made us unpleasant to be around. We all ran to where it was not safe to run. We all played with our genitals in sight of some prude. Someone made it our fault, and we believed them until we could blame them.

Check this out by thinking about your life today. How much of what you are unhappy about will cause you to blame yourself or to blame another? Maybe this paradigm only fits some of your experiences, or maybe the parts where it doesn't seem to fit consciously fall into the category of fits that are unconscious. It's rare to even bump against another person without each claiming or projecting fault.

Oftentimes the blame isn't over the fact itself but is over the emotions we experience in regard to the fact. Being told to not worry, to not be sad, to forgive, to KEEP CALM AND CARRY ON, and to think what Jesus would do are all messages that others give us to make us feel we aren't what we should be until we can feel differently. It's just a modification from the infantile idea that we must do differently.

Try to estimate what percentage of advertising strives to make the consumer see a need to have more, look better, be more, be safer or in some way tries to make the target of the ad feel not adequate with what they have or are. Or how about the said and unsaid messages we get from teachers, clergy, spouses, offspring, neighbors, doctors, salespeople, ad infinitum, and even our pets! How often does such make you find some fault with the advertiser or advisor if you don't find fault with yourself? Repeat—BS says that if anything is less than what you want, you will feel inadequate unless (SOB) the other has the inadequacy. It's one or the other, or maybe it's in the middle of the tilt, but if there is ill feeling, unmet wishes, or grief, it is somewhere on the tilt of that balance scale.

As we grow up, we are fed all kinds of myths, but most of them are reversed as we mature. We are taught to believe in fairness. We may be taught a religion. We might be taught to be racist. We were once taught people with penises go out into the world to make their fortune. Those without penises stay home, clean, and cook. That was back in the era in which Donald Trump said America was great! None of these messages will ever have the power of the BS because they were taught much later, often within the period of the past memory of the adult. The later a lie is taught, the easier it is to reject. About equally important, our adult world often will seek to modify those beliefs. Adulthood will really not let you believe in Santa Claus, may attempt to change your religion, will try to educate you to not be racist, and will push toward an acceptance of women's equality in all areas, but it will, most unfortunately, never discourage your belief in good/bad, right/wrong, and the need for punishment; those things were instilled in the BS/SOB period of very early life.

The new sexual freedom of the last half century is great. We can all have more orgasms in more interesting ways and places if we want. But it fails to make us feel we don't need to be better than we are, and it does little to lower the expectation that it is either our fault or our mate's fault if it doesn't turn out the way we want. And, especially in America, necessary cautions about consequences are much less emphasized than the infantile ideas of good and bad.

My first step to becoming a more skilled tennis player was to get a new grip on the racket. My first step to becoming a happier person is to get a grip on the idea that the Original Bullshit and the Shift of Blame need to go the way of fairy tales. The belief we should be better than we are has to go nest with Mother Goose—equally so the idea that anyone else should be better than they are.

Infants can't handle a glass of milk because they aren't yet toddlers. Wait a minute, I still spill milk! The model airplane fell apart because I tried to make it, unknowingly, a while before I had the needed skills. It was neither my fault nor another's fault. Thinking like this helps to pull us into the future with excitement. Believing BS and the SOB blocks our happiness, corrupts our governments, perverts our religions, and makes less effective our attempts to fight crime, educate our children, and provide or receive medical care.

5

You Can't Take the Infant Out of the Adult

WE WON'T EVER get over it. If steel, glass, plastic, leather, and rubber get run through a Ford factory, it will be a Ford forever. It might be nice if during its useful life we could turn our Buick into a Bentley, our Pinto into a Porsche, but it ain't gonna happen. We can modify it into an imitation of another, but then we just have a custom-bodied Pinto that is a Porsche look-alike. It's still shit in every aspect that we did not specifically, and with great expense and trouble, pay attention to altering. What gets laid down at the beginning of life is the corner-stone for as long as the edifice (psyche) shall exist. But what mis-engineering we can see and fix does improve the product.

Another way of saying this is if a woman who speaks only English moves to France as an adult and gains some proficiency in French, she will probably scream, "Help!" rather than, *"Aidez-moi!"* should the taxi in which she is riding overturn on the Champs Élysées. Don't ar-gue about at what point the new language imprints in the mind. Just accept the fact that what

31

we learned first is always in there and at times of stress comes out. Adults who have spoken a new language for decades may be found to be speaking only their native tongue after a severe enough brain injury. Likewise, what ever we learn about the absurdity of thinking in wrong and right as adults, it will come out in times of enough stress that we are right back to accusing and blaming.

We'll always be fearing shame, blame, guilt, or fear itself. Equally obnoxious are beliefs in pride, righteousness, virtue, and goodness. If a Ford will always be a Ford, if a person who learns to think in childhood will always have infantile ideas central in him, why do the work that I do? For two reasons: first, children to come can have better ideas engineered into them—not in infancy but in and after childhood; and second, those of us who have lived most of our lives in this darkness can learn to open our eyes to the light. There is a reason to understand the engineering of Porsches, even if we are, and will continue to breed, Fords. Even if I got my ideas in infancy and my children and grandchildren did also, there is still a point in understanding what adulthood is all about. We will be happier to stop going through life as adults with the minds of infants when it comes to right and wrong; to a large extent we are able to master that.

A simpler answer is merely that tennis lessons do bring more fun to the game even if our playing is never flawless. The more we learn to give up the effects of that Original BS that was done to us, the happier and healthier we can become even if we die someday with much Ford or Buick still in us. The frog that jumps one half of the way to the pond on every jump will never get in the water, but it surely will get close, and close is good enough; it's as happy as we can get.

We may alter or reject or accept variants to what rules we were taught as children, but the basic infantile concept that there is such a thing as wrong or right, good or bad doesn't get the same re-examination, and it should. Even though we can't rear a child without their adopting right/wrong thinking, we can begin to teach in later childhood that it is a myth, no more truth than Tigger and Roo and Winnie the Pooh.

Conflicted emotions do not cause problems–symptoms. Conflicts over emotions do. We were all taught to feel badly about ourselves whenever we experienced sadness, anger, hate, grief, or fear. One must learn to experience those true emotions free of self-doubt in order to be a happier person. Anxiety, depression, guilt, shame, worry, regret, and angst are all symptoms that come from being conflicted over the true emotions of fear and sadness and rob us of happiness and health because we were so conditioned from infancy to hate or blame ourselves when we were unhappy. Anyone can learn to be happier and mentally healthier. But just like you have to know the proper grip of the tennis racket, you also must stop seeing yourself or others as good or bad, right or wrong.

It is tempting to doubt my contention that we are conditioned to feel badly about ourselves when we feel sad or afraid, and it is more tempting to doubt my contention that we need not feel badly about ourselves when we feel anger and hatred. Feeling the conflicting emotions of love and hate, confidence and fear, and joy and grief doesn't cause symptoms, but debasing oneself for having such conflicts does.

Pavlov's dog stopped secreting stomach acid to the sound of the bell sometime after Pavlov stopped giving the dog food at the sound of the bell. To the extent that one really works at it, the adult can stop secreting unhappiness at the sound of misfortune by not bringing shame and blame to the sound of grief or anger.

"I am not what happened to me,
I am what I choose to become."

CARL JUNG

6

Eating from the Tree of Knowledge Is not Sin

I PROMISED to explain in chapter 6 my contention there are no such things as right and wrong and good and bad, and–in the way that I mean it–this contention doesn't disagree with most theology. When I explain myself, the concept will seem obvious but inane. One could benefit from what I am saying about happiness even if this strange idea were never proposed, but one's understanding would be superficial. In my effort to alleviate anxiety, depression, worry, guilt, and shame, I find the concept that there is no such thing as good or bad to be so helpful that I use it despite the initial disruptiveness of doing so.

I hate to break it to you, but bad or good didn't happen if I kill you. You getting dead is what happened! You can like or dislike that, but badness or goodness is only a statement of whether one is for or against you being dead. What goes against all of society's norms is what all of society doesn't like. Anything we call wrong or bad is nothing more than something inconvenient or unpleasant to us. If we search for a philosophical unity in defining good or bad, we're merely looking for what everyone would agree they do or don't like. If we believed in a god who wanted the earth to be protected from overpopulation, Adolph Hitler and Joseph Stalin would appear to some as among the best of men, modern-day Noahs out to save their own while the others got offed.

Let's understand this from an evolutionary perspective. When the Event took place fifteen billion years ago, was it good or bad that it did? Is it good or bad that anything exists? Was it good or bad that the earth's axis is tilted from the sun? When the dinosaurs roamed the earth, was there morality? Were the brontosauri good because they didn't eat other animals, and were T. Rex bad because they did? Ten thousand millennia later, were ethics invented when mammals reached a certain point?

Some think only people can be bad; others think their dog can be bad. A common concept is badness or goodness can reside in humans but not lower animals. Some would see for such ideas there are no data. Did something monumental emerge in the cosmos called *bad* when Arthur C. Clarke's ape picked up the stick? Or did it have to await Stanley Kubrick's making of the movie for bad to happen? Good and bad did not evolve at Olduvai Gorge. In fact, they never evolved at all.

Was your ex-spouse evil in some way the rats that carried the fleas that carried the bacteria that caused the Black Death were not? Or was the pathogen in the air conditioning ducts in the Bellevue-Stratford Hotel that caused Legionnaires' Disease morally different, ethically different, good or bad different than the virus that causes AIDS or the necessary bacteria in our bowels without which our bodies would not process food?

Am I bad when I swat a fly? Are we bad if we wipe out the last of a species, or of our own species? Was it bad when mankind killed off the smallpox virus? Is there evil in a child with a different number of digits than twenty? Which is better, a left-handed child or a right-handed child? Is there good or bad in an infant with a hole in the septum of his heart? What if he's born with the stigma of a genetic trisomy? Does this involve good or evil? What if one's brain chemistry causes anxious suffering in new situations or makes one crave stimulation beyond what is available in the milieu? Is one good or bad to be conservative or liberal or hyperactive? What if one's brain is wired such that normal emotions are missing? Is it possible Jeffrey Dahmer and Ted Bundy were not bad even though they were dangerous? Do we protect ourselves from rattlesnakes because they are evil or because they are dangerous? Do we kill them (rattler or pervert) to protect ourselves or to punish them for being bad? I write this most humbly because I am not a philosopher and do not pretend to be an intellectual, but it seems to me so much happier to go through life without useless concepts of good or evil and to get street smart as to what is dangerous and what is not and how to know the difference and protect ourselves and those we love.

Serial killers are not different from us because they have badness and we have goodness. They are different from us because they are different from us. An animal that eats noxious vermin is not more good than an animal that eats children lost in the woods. They are different animals.

I don't like serial killers. I don't like the West Nile Virus. I'd like to eliminate or prevent the breeding of serial killers and the West Nile Virus, but I don't attribute good or bad to either.

I do believe evil exists, as does beauty and a whole host of words used to describe concepts or objects or events, but evil and beauty are not objects or events in themselves. They are language constructs. They are defined by our own perspective to allow us to communicate with others. They are not tangible, real objects. They are no more real than are the Tooth Fairy, Santa Claus, Father Time, Baby New Year or the Easter Bunny. The use of those words does not give substance to any belief in some sort of gooey substance called *badness* that invades the beings whose behavior we do not countenance.

If one believes in Satan or a devil and sin, nothing is really changed; it's just kicked back one level. One must still understand the sinner was a normal, perfect human on which the devil did his work. You can't believe all evil comes from Satan and then believe somehow the human was already bad as it encountered Satan. Would you really believe Eve was in some way bad and that was why she was vulnerable before she encountered the serpent? If so, from where came that flaw before she met the devil? If I were to believe she was perfect without some vulnerability before she met the serpent, I would not be able to fault her. OK, that leaves us with the devil being bad. Here we are on a merry-go-round of inane truisms. Let's not say that the devil was supposed to be good; if he were, then he's a bad devil. (And isn't that a good devil—to be bad?) Now I understand the belief that man can't understand the ways of God, but this whole paragraph is inane.

How interesting that in the creation myth, sin began with eating from the Tree of Knowledge.

When Robert Oppenheimer fired off Gadget on July 16, 1945, there floated through his mind a line from the *Bhagavad Gita,* "I am become death, the shatterer of worlds." I maintain that if one were to look at the history of civilization as being modeled on a human life span, then that predawn blast in the New Mexico desert would be symbolized by an adolescent getting the car keys. From that instant on, civilization could destroy itself or could accomplish beyond all previous imagination. My opinion that Trinity was the most dramatic event in the history of mankind never made me see it as bad or good. Only Rick Santorum or the most controlling tsar or pope or parent could see the acquiring of knowledge as bad in itself.

I can teach you how to be a happier person if you are willing to act and think as if good, bad, right, and wrong don't exist when you face yourself and behave toward your fellow animals, *Homo sapiens* and other species.

I used the following example with patients; they told me they found it helpful. It goes like this: I'm downhill skiing and wrap my leg around a fir tree. My tibia snaps and cuts through the tissues of my leg, and my zillion-dollar Bogner ski pants are shredded and bloody. Blood pools in the snow. I pass out from the pain as I piss my pants. I awake to see you standing there asking me what is wrong with my leg. I retort there is absolutely nothing wrong with my leg. It is doing exactly what any perfect leg does when you wrap it around a tree when skiing as out of control as I was a moment, an eternity, ago. Whether there is something wrong with my leg is a moot issue. Even if I die from blood loss or the shock of the pain, it is just not true there is anything wrong or bad—or even imperfect—in that leg. What we need to be concerned with is stopping the bleeding and then getting me to an operating room and in the hands of a skilled orthopedic surgeon. A little something for the pain might be nice as well. But we don't need to blame the leg or to see it as deficient in any way.

But if some human gets wrapped around not yet understood forces and spills some gore, society doesn't get concerned with fixing or even discovering the problem. It is preoccupied with punishing. We will spend fortunes trying to decide if someone who is deadly is bad enough that we get to kill him or if he's not quite that bad so we have to feed and house him and medically treat him in a prison somewhere forever. There is no question he is so dangerous that he can't be allowed to be in society. The multimillion-dollar question (actually) is only how bad he is. I don't claim to know the answer to what we should do with people who are dangerous to others. I do not find it something I expect of myself to figure out what criminologists haven't figured out. I am glad they are now concerning themselves with what their disciplines can be learning to do to protect us from dangerous people instead of microscopically trying to divine the amount of good or bad that is in each human sample. Academia does seem to be ahead of our courts on that one.

I have been involved in trials and jury selections in cases of first-degree murder with special circumstances and was astounded to actually hear the officers of the court arguing if the offenders were bad enough that we're justified in killing them or if there were some redeeming protons and electrons in the condemned that should spare them from such extermination. They were not arguing about escape risk, some eventual parole, or even about cost of detention versus execution. They weren't even concerned with the idea of a wrongful conviction. They were arguing about how bad was the cold-blooded murderer.

We'd have a happier society if we could learn what kinds of differences in mind function cause some people to be dangerous and how we could protect ourselves from them. There is wasted unhappiness in our world because we have to see some people as better, more good, more bad, worse, more evil, more *et cetera* than ourselves. I am not so naive as to believe mankind will ever be able to figure out all of the differences between dangerous and non-dangerous persons (or politicians), but I think we should aver those differences do exist.

So far in the twenty-first century AD, the at-risk ones are free to roam society and do whatever dangerous thing they want to do. After they have done their harm, then we call them bad and kill them. I'm not arguing for prior restraint. I am arguing for ongoing curiosity, understanding, research, and the scientific method of always wondering more and trying to learn more instead of assuming they are bad and we are good and that's it.

Let's face this fact: Acts of God are acts of a god until we learn something new, then they stop being acts of a god. No longer do educated people see a god's retribution in earthquakes, hurricanes, eclipses, or northern lights. Our understanding of climatology is now such that no one believes our society's rudimentary acceptance of homosexuals can cause hurricanes—no one except some who pretend to have very rigid senses of right and wrong that they can sell to ignorant masses for their own profit. Likewise, what was earlier thought of as bad became something else when we learned that children have neurological conditions resulting in attention deficit disorder, autism, or epilepsy. Now those children are no longer bad.

Left-handedness was once considered bad—left-handed persons were thought to be sinister (Latin: sinister—left, wrong, unfavorable, on the left hand, on the left side, perverse), and lefties were punished and bullied in preposterous attempts at forced reassignment of handedness. The bad went away when neuroanatomy revealed lateral dominance of the brain. A century ago, intelligent people stopped seeing left-handedness as a sign of a devil or of evil; in this century, the same can be said for sexual preference differences. In the duration of my career, homosexuality has gone from being an evil to a mental illness then back again to being an evil and on to being a difference of a minority, like left-handedness. For a professional today to try to change sexual orientation is seen as wrongheaded—though far more harmful—as it once was to try to alter handedness.

It was inconceivable a few moments (centuries) ago that the witches being hanged in America or burned in Europe were anything other than evil. Since then we have found other explanations for the innocent behaviors that raised accusations. In the news at this time are discoveries that are changing our minds about why people are obsessive-compulsive, conservative or liberal, and believers or doubters. I firmly believe long after you and I are dead there will be an entirely different explanation of serial killers, of Charles Ponzi, of defiant children, and of people who drink thirty-two-ounce sodas.

There are people out there in the headlines, prominent in political parties, and leading our secular and religious organizations who have ideas just as poorly developed as the dogmatic tenets of the witch hangers. Every time there is a human tragedy caused by a violent person, those idiots are out of their minds, as well as out of their expertise, pontificating about what this means about God and good and devils and evil, and they have no idea whatsoever what causes human actions.

I do not pretend to be preeminent, but it is time to just give up on good/bad and right/wrong. We don't need to be first taught we are bad and then taught we need to be forgiven, saved, redeemed, or punished. The good news (gospel) of salvation is that nobody needs it.

I maintain there is nothing bad in anyone. Some people are bigots and others understand, just like some snakes are poisonous and others are not. It is not a flaw in an adder for it to be venomous. It is not a flaw in a stupid person to be stupid. A person can be perfectly stupid just like a snake can be perfectly toxic. We do need to learn which snakes we can safely pet and which persons we can safely face. If a religious person believes all humans have sinned, how can he aver that to have done so makes one a bad human?

One of the many things unfortunate about the effects of the Original BS is it forces us to be far too dependent on externals for our view of ourselves. We were taught if the others around us like what we do, we are good. If they don't, we're bad. We then think like that for the rest of our lives unless we are Born Again, understanding it only comes from misunderstanding, and do what we can about it as adults.

I have had patients who have said they were never given messages about the need to be better—their parents were far too loving to have done such. This reminds me of my twelve-year-old patient who protested her parents would have never been so nasty as to have engaged in sex. She was just too young at the time of her conception to recall it. Good/bad and wrong/right messages happen before one is old enough to remember. The sooner it stops, the better off is the child, to be sure. But starting with being weaned from the breast, learning to use a spoon, getting potty-trained, or being put to bed in the crib, any infant gets and incorporates a false core message it must become better than it is.

The power of the parents (I'm including here, of course, parent substitutes of every ilk—in the case of Romulus and his twin it was a wolf, for Tarzan it was an ape) over the ideas which are at the very core of adults-to-be is just beyond all understanding. We say, "Oh, yes," but the more one understands, the more one realizes it can't be fully understood.

In the Middle Ages, a student approached a teacher to learn about the natural world. The teacher gave the student a dead fish and told him to take the fish and learn from it all that he could. The student returned in five minutes and told the teacher what he had learned. The teacher sent him away again with the same instruction. The student returned after an hour with far more observations. The teacher repeated the instruction, and the student returned months later with still more knowledge. The teacher repeated the instruction yet again, and the student is still out studying the fish.

Our knowledge of how our characters are shaped is like the knowledge of the fish that is still being studied. We continually examine how we know what we think we know, and the more we know, the more we know we don't know. We see children cry for their parents and cling to them in the emergency room where they are being treated for their injuries as their parents who have beaten them are led off to the jailhouse for child abuse. The child is welded to how he is parented with no ability to distinguish abuse or errors or lies from what is rational long before he develops memories which are part of his adult thinking.

Many religious patients at first rejected my ideas that there is no good/bad, right/wrong. I would tell them that we use those words, properly, to label things as being what we do like or don't like. They would rightly object on the basis of their belief in a divine sense of good and evil. I would ask them to understand there was really no difference between what I was saying and their beliefs by showing them that what they were calling sin, I was calling those acts which would separate them from God—good if they want to be separated from God, bad only if they don't want to be separated from God. With that understanding, we could be unified in our discussions. Righteousness is bad if you want to be removed from the god in which you believe.

In the introduction to this book, I claimed my ideas were accepted by priests and ministers as being compatible with their theology, and yet I am denying the existence of sin and rejecting any need for salvation. I promised that I would elucidate this contention. Many of them believe that every human has sinned and is in need of salvation to avoid eternal damnation. I maintain that every human needs vitamin D to avoid rickets. There is nothing wrong with a person for needing vitamin D and those theologians can come to accept the idea that, in this sense, there is nothing wrong with an individual for needing salvation. Everything I have to say about the happiness that is to come from accepting oneself unconditionally does not gainsay that all have sinned and need salvation any more than that all have incompetent bones without vitamin D. I don't share their belief in sin and salvation, but they have come to see that we can all agree that any truly universal trait of mankind doesn't presage any need for any person to feel inadequate or to accept oneself only conditionally. If sin is seen as a universal of all mankind, then no individual needs to feel personally guilty for being a sinner any more than they might feel physically defective for needing that vitamin.

There are tools to be described in this book that will help readers to be healthier and happier even if they cannot buy every point I'm making, but the more that one can give up believing in right/wrong and good/bad, the easier will be the journey. I know it's not possible to think of a Himmler as not being bad, but remember in our own nation's history, one-quarter of the population at one time saw Abraham Lincoln as unmitigated evil. It's plain to us today to see those who saw him as evil as themselves evil for enslaving fellow men, but those rebels saw themselves as godly men who worshipped in church as they profited and became wealthy by twisting doctrine while blinded by their self interest. Even though it complicates how we see Mr. Lincoln, the US Constitution at the time of the Civil War recognized the right of each state to peacefully withdraw from the union at its own will. No Confederate leader was ever brought to trial for treason because such a trial would have exposed the constitutional legality of secession. One familiar with the magnitude of the horrors of that war might easily conclude that Mr. Lincoln was the greatest war criminal in history up until his time.

Before we leave this discussion of BS and SOBs and the idea that knowledge or its lack cannot be sin, I want to address head on the objections of those who say that men and women will be inadequately socialized and harmful to each other if their inner nature is not modified by rules, shame, and guilt. There are religious people who teach man is bad and must be saved. Whenever I speak about guilt, punishment, and shame always being inappropriate, even atheists have objections because of their fear that their children may be bad if they aren't taught to not be bad. Most atheists are too religious. They are basing this fallacy on a system of good and bad that is unsupported by anything other than belief (faith!).

Humans absolutely depend on being loved for life itself in the beginning. No child reaches any stage of development unless it is cared for by another human (Remus, his twin, and Tarzan excepted). Monkeys will not thrive if they are cared for by machines. The experiment which demonstrated this in rhesus macaques (Harry Harlow) cannot be repeated with human infants for obvious ethical reasons, but I see no reasonable doubt that children need love to develop. Our personalities take form before our bodies can exist outside a loving nurture. Actually, surprising as it may seem, even some adults need love! Those who equate atheism with bad are ignorant of the implications of this. Belief in a god is not necessary in order for a human to be humane. I am not arguing for the atheists or agnostics. I am averring that religious people can believe what they do without needing to see people who don't as being bad. Men become harmful to each other as the result of the BS and the SOB; absent that, the problems that society tries to modify with shame, guilt, and punishment would not exist. Exceptions to this are psychotics or sociopaths who are not made safe by any moral teaching anyway.

When one looks at Ivan the Terrible, it's easy to believe in evil. When the ancients felt the earth move or saw volcanoes erupt, it was just as obvious for them to attribute this to the displeasure of the gods. One does not have to believe in the gods to understand geological marvels today, and one doesn't have to believe in evil to explain Ivan.

There are biological variations in all parts of the body and in all species of living things. These can be explained on a basis other than good or bad. The variations may explain absence of pigment, extra toes, two-headed snakes, and brain aberrations that cause altered function. Couple this with a world in which billions of persons were taught the BS and SOB of infancy and it's to be expected that a number of humans will be sociopaths. It does not depend on evil and good to explain a Rodrigo Borgia, Saddam Hussein, or Lee Harvey Oswald any more than a Mozart, Michael Phelps, or Alan Turing.

"Puritanism:
The haunting fear that someone,
somewhere may be happy."

H. L. MENCKEN

7

Adultery Is More Fun Than Infancy

JUST ABOUT EVERYONE educated in the Western world knows Dr. Freud saw the mind as housing the ego, id, and super-ego. What is less talked about is the super-ego becomes subservient to the ego as much as the subject advances into adulthood. If one were fully adult, the super-ego would cease to exist; its functions would be assumed by the ego.

That is what I hated about academic psychiatry. Why not just say that to the extent one grows up, one thinks for oneself and doesn't act on the basis of what one was taught as an infant by those living in a different era? Those who tell us we should listen to our conscience—that still, small voice—are encouraging us to stay infants. All that voice is about is the BS message, which should be waning about the time we find hair growing in our axillae.

This chapter proclaims life is happier at those rare moments when we can think as adults. If I'm doing what my conscience tells me, I'm acting as an infant. If I'm deciding what I want to do on the basis of with what consequences I choose to live, I am an adult for that moment. This triggers a philosophical debate over whether one really is ever free to do this. I'm not going to go there. If mankind has not solved the issue of free will versus determinism, then neither will I. To whatever extent I am able, I'm happier when I'm not bound by the need to be better than I am or blame another but am free to do as I wish with the only condition being that I have to live with the consequences of my actions. I can't ever really know the consequences of my actions; that is admittedly a problem. (When a historian was recently asked what were the consequences of the French Revolution, he replied, "It's too soon to know.") But that problem is not solved by the childish notion that I can avoid ill by being not fully responsible for my behavior because I'm instead listening to my conscience. I can't cop out by obeying and then blaming the one whom I'm obeying. We heard enough of that at Nuremberg over seventy years ago.

WWJD might be a useful goad in organizing my thoughts about an upcoming decision, but accepting what my caretaker might have told me when I was too young to have the wisdom of today is not—at least without making it subservient to what I now think. As an adult, I will recognize that teachers, magazines, books, mates, friends, and even my dog will know things I don't. Of course, it is wise to drink at the fountain of their knowledge, but as an adult I make the decision of what it is I'm going to ingest.

About four decades ago, I was on the verge of doing something that a feeling inside of me told me I must not do. I was willing to live with the consequences of what I was going to do, and I wanted it done. I started wondering from whence came my discomfort. After a quick reality and memory check, I remembered when I was a grade schooler my mother had told me I must never do what I was about to do. Then I began to think about whether the twenty-nine-year-old, uneducated woman who was my mother in 1946 should be making decisions for a thirty-five-year-old man with twenty-five years of schooling who was living in 1976 about what he was going to do in 1976. I will never be fully grown up and to that extent will never be free of those old influences. And—until I become prescient—I will never be sure of the consequences of any actions. But I still should be responsible for myself and make my decisions on the best of what I've got now, not cop out and irresponsibly just obey that twenty-nine-year-old who lived decades earlier.

Here's a better one: when I was a child, my parents were socially insecure. My father was a just-graduated physician. They were from poor backgrounds, and neither had any experience in dealing with middle-class prosperity such as was the case with the people then in their

46

milieu. It was probably in response to an elementary school classmate's birthday party invitation coupled with some degree of her own inferiority complex that my mother told me when I get an invitation, I must decline. They were inviting me just to be nice, not because they wanted me to come. When they were nice enough to invite me, I mustn't be rude enough to actually accept. Granted the words used here are those of an adult–I remember the message and the hurt, not the vocabulary. Now, here's the fun part. In my seventies, I have more wonderful, loving friends than I ever thought possible. Many have been my closest treasures for decades. I adore them and am in awe at my good fortune. I trust them explicitly. I entertain a lot. Whenever one of them invites me to anything, my mother's message from seven decades ago must be consciously neutralized before I can even think about what I am being invited to. Now the crucial thing is that I am left with a far more lingering invite-phobia than my mother experienced. She accepted this bit of nonsense as a young adult. It was taught to me in early childhood. It was more deeply rooted in me than it was in her because of the early age at which I was exposed to the rubbish.

Of course, one cannot be born again. Obviously, I'm using this as a metaphor. My idea of the phrase to "be born again" would be to experience an adult level of responsibility, caring, loving, and knowing the consequences of behavior with a high degree of wisdom and intelligence while one gainsays the lies and misperceptions of infancy about right or wrong. This is accomplished by understanding what has been said in chapter 2 and forming a new life, a new me, based on the adult understanding there is no right/wrong and no good/bad.

If someone accuses me of having hurt them, I would prefer to experience sadness that they are hurt, perhaps I do what I can to aid them or make restitution, but they have no power to make me feel there is something wrong with me. That hurt may have happened because I was an idiot, careless, thinking only of myself, or not using common sense. Well, I know that I'm not all grown up yet, and this will make me, in the next instant, less hurtful than I was a second ago, but this is what it is to be human. How "bad" I am is not the point; the point is you were hurt. As I learn from this and become less hurtful, I needn't feel shame I wasn't more grown up a moment ago than I was a moment ago. I will turn my attention to helping you and expressing sadness you were hurt and sadness I hurt you instead of wallowing in guilt and apology and distracting you from your pain with attempts to get you to forgive me.

I want to be equally immune to pride. If someone praises me, I'm aware I just encountered one of the people in the world who likes what I did, fully aware there are also those out there who do not like what I did. If I'm insulted, I just learned I'm in the vicinity of an insulter. If I lose a foot race, I realize the guy out there who can run faster than I showed up. If I win, I realize he did not show up. In the first case I'm sad I lost the race; in the second case I'm happy I won, but I do not feel better or worse about myself. This is what it is to be adult.

What if I could conduct my romances thrilled if the one I love loves me, saddened if the one I love does not love me, but immune from feeling better or worse about myself in either case? Imagine finding myself to have been petty, cruel, and niggardly to the extent of saddening another and reflexly saddening myself. Next, I grieve I wasn't more grown up than I was at that moment, then I learn from the experience. Next I make the effort and change my behavior, seeing myself as advancing away from infancy and toward adulthood for doing so.

Mazda used to make a car called the GLC (an acronym for Great Little Car). I used this as a mnemonic in my work, teaching patients what we jokingly referred to as Mazda therapy. When one does something for which one would previously have felt shame, guilt, or remorse, one is Born Again when one will instead Grieve, Learn, and Change. That process makes for a happier adult than the one who feels the more infantile shame or guilt. Growth is inhibited by guilt or shame, spurred by a desire to learn and change.

In the sense of my vocabulary in writing this book (I agree that I am teaching from a very specialized lexicon, which I made up), adults feel joy, happiness, sadness, anger, and fear while children of any age feel pride, worry, depression, shame, and anxiety. Better said would be, Born Agains feel the former while those still believing BS and living with the SOB feel the latter.

I've wanted to write a movie scene demonstrating how bizarre infancy would be if the infant could think as an adult. Here's the scene: Two-Year-Old is in the high chair in the kitchen. Mother (yes, she does have a lot to learn, too) hands the child a glass of milk, which Two-Year-Old throws on the floor. Mother lovingly tells Two-Year-Old to try to be a little more careful, or she scolds Two-Year-Old for throwing the glass on the floor, or she bops the kid upside the head, or she knocks over the high chair and stomps on the two-year-old. In any of these cases, Two-Year-Old looks at Mother and says, "Mom, I know you're tired; you've had an exhausting day. I'm saddened by the fact I've made your day more complicated. I wish the glass were not broken, milk weren't running across the floor and under the refrigerator, and milk didn't cost so much. I also wish I could have consumed that milk, because I am hungry. But I'm not going to allow you to make me feel badly about the fact that I don't know yet how to control a glass of milk. If you wanted me to behave today like a three-year-old you should have birthed me a year earlier than you did! You didn't, so I'm behaving like a two-year-old. This will be one of the experiences which will go into making me a person in the future who spills less." This, by the way, is equally relevant whether the child deposits the glass upon the floor through lack of coordination or through defiance.

I know there are challenges to my ideas on the above subjects, and I don't believe I'm any more right than those who espouse those challenges. Huh? What am I saying? I'm saying on the path of becoming happier adults, we are aided by giving up the concept we are worse than those who don't like us unless we are better than those who don't like us–giving up that we can like ourselves better if those who like us are in the majority than we can if those who like us are in the minority.

How tragic that we fear all of our lives we will be, or that others will see us as being, wrong. Equally tragic is seeing oneself as being right.

I happen to be very aware of style when it comes to furnishing my home. It has a certain look, and I enjoy that look. It, the style, is pretty minimalistic. I get joy out of seeing how few things I can live with and how they all interplay. But that does not make for anything good or better than the homes of those who love lots of La-Z-Boys and tchotchkes all over the place. I'm happier having what I want and enjoying others who have what they want if I don't have inferiority that is infancy-bred for which I need to compensate by seeing people who care more about comfort than I as being boobs. By the way, I enjoy small-breasted-women and do so more if I don't fabricate some psychological defect to be in women who get augmented.

The other person can only tell you about the other person. He cannot tell you about yourself. If you make fun of my singing, I have learned nothing about my being tone deaf. I've only learned about your tastes and manners. I'm happy to admit I may not know what I've learned at that, but your behavior is about you, not about me. If I clumsily bump into a man who then decks me for not showing him more deference, I just learned I bumped into an asshole–that said with an apology to a perfectly good part of the body for using it as a demeaning reference. I already knew I was clumsy.

Let's go a step further. What if I think I can sing well enough to get people to pay me to sing, and everyone tells me I can't sing? Am I claiming that I should go right on believing I can sing well enough to make my living singing? Sure, I am. But I will soon learn no one is going to pay me to sing or even stick around if I try to sing. I will learn something about them. Then, I get to do what I want to do with what I've learned about them. If I want to go on singing for the dog, I needn't feel shame, or maybe I'll lip sync; perhaps I would be happier to try something else. I'm writing this book because I want to write it. The fact no one may buy it will teach me about the public and the market. Were it to become a best seller, it wouldn't make me think I'm a writer.

While parking, I once tapped the bumper of the car parked in front of my space with its ass end protruding five feet into my space, which made my parking in the only available space an arduous task. After the slightest kiss of the rubber parts of our automobiles, I noticed a woman sitting in the other car–sitting in the other car for a microsecond before she descended upon me like a wicked witch of a tornado. After she had spun beyond control and then sputtered out, I looked up and apologized for upsetting her and expressed the hope I had not put a mark on her car–the lack of which, of course, was obvious to both of us. A friend who noticed the transaction was amazed at my response and amazed I did not sound sarcastic. Well, there was nothing to be amazed about and nothing to be sarcastic about. An emotionally fragile woman had been traumatized that she was not a princess and her car was not Cinderella's pumpkin coach. I was glad I had not hurt her car and sad I had met her. The incompetence of her parking was irrelevant to me, as was what she thought of me. She was doing the best she could do at that instant, and I respected that. I had no reason to blame her or to try to put her in her place for her behavior or point out her lack of parking expertise, because I had no reason to compensate for blaming myself. Had I needed to do so, it would have been a much less happy day for me. It's more fun to be adult than infant.

I told a raunchy joke in a place I felt such a joke to be appropriate. In fact, the agenda was to see who could tell the raunchiest joke. I probably would have won the contest except I was devastated when someone pointed out that my joke was highly offensive to anyone who had ever been the subject of a particular type of childhood molestation. How could a psychiatrist . . . ? How could I have been so blind to the offensive nature of my joke to that subset of the population? I felt depressed until I remembered what I always tried to teach my patients. At that moment I really was that dumb, that blind. I needed that experience to make me wiser in the next moment. There was no shame in not having learned that particular lesson before I learned it. Now, that said, I have to go further and take total responsibility. The environment of that raunchy joke contest was not responsible for drawing me into telling my little anecdote. The telling of that tale tells me only about me. I learned something about my own blindness. I grieved I hadn't seen it sooner. And I'll not tell that joke in public again.

The behavior of the other persons only tells me about them. My detractors at the joke contest probably revealed that a lot of them had been molested. Rather than using that as an excuse for why I offended them, I see it as further reason for my sadness and resolve to delete that joke. My behavior only tells me about me. If you step on my foot and I shove you, I shove you only because I am rude and stupid. If I had my foot close enough to you for you to step on it, I am responsible for that, too.

I have had the rich, wonderful experience of knowing several individuals who lived well into their nineties and still were bright and wise. They, those oldsters, really have it together—at least the ones I have known. They were not subject to intimidation. They could not be seduced. They'd say exactly what they meant without needless insult or a desire to hurt anyone. A favorite vignette took place when Lucile (you will read a lot more about her soon), at about the age of eighty-nine, first visited my stylish, minimalist home and could find no piece of furniture which invited her to sit. She looked at the Corbusier, Rietveld, van der Rohe, and Breuer and then asked me, "David, if you were going to sit someplace for a long time, which chair would you choose." It became a favorite joke about my house. I laughed and told her, "Lucile, the chairs are all meant to be looked at, not sat in." I don't remember how we resolved the situation. I remember she was not going to insult me or quietly make herself uncomfortable.

A ninety-six-year-old friend of mine was doing her laundry one Easter morning in the community facility of a Christian retirement home where she lived. She was discovered by the wife of the retired minister who ran the place and challenged, "Is this the way you celebrate the day of the resurrection of Our Lord?" My friend straightened the posture of her four-foot-eight, shrunken, ancient body and announced, "Yes." End of story. No need for any excuse or apology and no need to insult the crone.

I was talking to a younger man about how I marveled at the wisdom and unflappability of those elderly persons, the ones who remained sharp and were free from dementia. My friend said, "Yes, they just don't care anymore." I disagreed. I think "caring" is not the quality they have shed. They have rid themselves of ideas that anyone can make them wrong or right or that they are better than anyone else, so they no longer need to see others as wrong. Many younger friends chide me over my lack of comfortable chairs; Lucile just wanted to know where to sit. My laundering friend just wanted to get her clothes clean. There was no inhibition based on any fear of anyone making her feel guilt.

A middle-aged woman, Melanie, came to see me because of anxiety caused by her employment and depression over marital stress. We worked with the above concepts–no job outcome was going to cause her to lessen her sense of self even if it caused her to get fired. No marital consequence could cause her to blame herself even if it did teach her to change her behavior. She did well in therapy and embraced what she needed to embrace to become much less anxious and depressed. One day, Melanie came in with a rather amazing application of those principles which neither of us would have foreseen. She told me that a few days prior, she remembered–for the first time in her adult life–having been molested by her grandfather when she was a small child. She seemed totally non-traumatized by the memory. When I inquired as to her equanimity over the whole thing, she replied that what the old goat had done really had nothing to do with her. Melanie had moved into adulthood on that issue, away from the BS and the SOB of infancy which would have caused her shame unless she could blame and punish the now-dead ancestor.

Of course, I believe in the Freudian concept of repression, but if one stops believing in shame and guilt, repressed memories emerge relatively non-traumatically and easily compared with the labor required to access those memories through the usual psychoanalytic process while one still believes in shame and guilt. If one can be so simplistic as to suggest that Freud taught us to not have shame over sex, I'd like to suggest it would have been better had he taught us to not have shame. Actually, I suspect he did, but the sex–not the shame–is what got the attention.

Another misconception of childhood, which is just accepted without examination, is that we will grow up. Children can't drive; adults can. Children have a different court system than do adults. Adults who act like narcissists are considered to be infantile. The problem is that we are 100 percent infants at the moment we are born. We get to be 100 percent as adult as we will ever be the moment that we die or lose our mind. In between those two extremes is a continual increase of maturation. But that is never explained. We believe we are supposed to know everything and have perfect judgment when we become adult. Well, it never happens and that is not something we should rue. We should just stop expecting complete maturity of ourselves and others.

People have taught me they can face without pause that they wet their diapers when they were infants but would have great embarrassment over an eliminatory accident as an adult. Well, that is certainly normal and would apply to us all, but it's a fact we never are adult enough to be 100 percent risk free of such events. I am a happier person when knowing if I pissed my pants a moment ago, however inconvenient, it is no more a cause for shame than it was when I was in preschool. And how happy I am it happens so much less often now.

The last part of infantile thinking I'd like to expose has to do with what we are taught as being the reason for life, for our existence. The happiest people are those who see life as being for no purpose. It just is, and you get to do with it what you want to do with it. Now, to understand this sentence one has to respect that I am including the consequence—long and short term—with the act, and I believe there is no instance wherein one is not responsible. I don't need to see work or doing for others or sacrifice or goodness as being what life is for. I can see life as being fun. It is more fun (and we will explore what appears to be the argument against this in future pages) to be loving, be responsible, pay one's bills, eat, stay warm and dry, keep the use of one's mind, maintain all of one's limbs, etc. But that doesn't deny the ultimate purpose of being kind to others, loving and protecting them, owning up, being able to provide for one's basic needs, maintaining mental health, behaving with a mind to safety, and working is still to have fun—to enjoy the life that we experience. If an evangelist were to shrink with horror at my supposition that life is for having fun, I'd remind him that in his system, loving God and doing what he needs to do to bring others to God is what he has decided he wants to do about what he believes, and he might as well have fun doing what he wants. There is no loss of integrity in the experience of joy.

The lessons I propose in this book can never be learned or applied completely. One of the definitions of a crisis is a circumstance wherein your best level of adulthood is inadequate to get you through, so you will either become more adult than you have ever been or will regress to a lower level of psychological maturation. We all will have crises forever. We all will come up against situations for which we are too infantile to have a desired result. We'd might as well get used to it and realize that the expectation we're all grown up is just one more absurdity.

I was taught by science teachers in high school who . . . ; well, let's just say I take some things they said as being "ain't necessarily so." I am not enough a chemist or physicist to vouch for the following story that my first chemistry teacher taught, but–true or not–it's a wonderful analogy for what this part of the book is proclaiming. He taught his classes that substances which exist in liquid form all contract when they cool and solidify except water at the freezing point. Added to this assertion was the point that water expanding when it freezes causes ice to float on water. If ice contracted like everything else, it would sink; the oceans would then freeze from the bottom up, and eventually, all of earth's water would be trapped in frozen seas surrounding lifeless continents. That would mean war is only possible because of the simple fact that H2O expands as it freezes. Likewise love and birth and you and I only exist because of that expansion. Without that one peculiarity of water, there would never have been a tree or a unicorn or the Oscars or a kiss or a Tesla (either man or car). Life itself would not exist.

I'm using the fact of water expanding as it freezes and therefore changing everything as an analogy for the lesson that believing the BS of infancy has changed everything. Learning to live as an adult would fix everything that is of psychological origin if only everyone could do it all the time.

If humans didn't believe they need to be better, stronger, wiser, more powerful, more right, have more, and be superior to their peers, they could solve most of the present causes of the world's unhappiness. If I were able to grow up into an adulthood absent those same misconceptions, I would be likewise happier.

Lucile was ninety-two years of age when she was dining with me in a fine restaurant and made a *faux pas* over which most persons would feel embarrassment. Instead, she looked up with a smile and said, "Isn't it great that at my age I am still learning." Lucile had the ability to move on to a more advanced state of learning without feeling shame she hadn't already mastered it in her tenth decade of life.

I believe many readers will see nothing in part 1 of this book as other than mental masturbation. That's what I would think if I read such written by another writer and stopped at this point. Please don't. The subject of part 2 is how one can use this Born Again enlightenment to change those thoughts that bring unhappiness into those consistent with mental health. Part 3 is practical applications of playing with the new grip through the challenges of life. This is the stuff Kay wanted me to write.

END OF PART ONE

What Mary Said

WHAT MARY SAID TO ME WAS MORE POTENT in shaping my career as a psychotherapist than any single thing any teacher, writer, or colleague ever told me.

Mary was a woman in her mid-forties. She'd never found a long-term mate. She abused alcohol and drugs, was often suicidal, and was not a happy camper. Mary had been raised in Connecticut and treated as an adolescent and adult by some of the most famous psychiatrists in New York City. Her family had enough money to have spent on her treatment what would buy a yacht. She had recently moved to California and was seeking a psychiatrist with whom to continue therapy. Mary had pretty much given up on ever becoming a happy or responsible person, but family and friends continued to push for more care, and she complied. I was intimidated when I learned she was coming to me—a very green physician who had been in practice only a few short years—after over twenty years of inpatient and outpatient (including psychoanalytic) treatment with some of the most prominent names in my profession.

During her first three months with me, Mary was often drunk, drugged, overdosed, or suicidal. I don't know any word to describe her generalized demeanor other than *bitch*. Early in treatment, she told me about a neurotic fear which caused a lot of her acting-out behavior. I responded that I shared the neurosis and had the same fear. She responded hostilely, perhaps thinking I was mocking her, and demanded to know how I thought I could help her if I had the same craziness as she did. My answer brought her around when I explained I could live happily and in peace with the fear, and I would help her to do the same.

Most of the time we had weekly, fifty-minute sessions. There were a few extra sessions for emergencies. After about a year she felt she was well; she was sober, off drugs, happy, making friends and thought she would stop therapy. I suggested—on the basis of her past history of never-ending treatment—that we might want to set a date a few months into the future at which we'd plan to stop therapy. It's amazing what benefit often comes in sessions when the patient knows the end of treatment is nigh; that advantage is lost with a termination that is unplanned.

We stopped therapy on the preset date, and she did not return. We had expended probably eighty-five sessions over eighteen months, and she left feeling she was a whole person. I wondered about her for years, always hopeful, but I couldn't believe we'd done something in those few sessions that had eluded all of her previous psychiatrists.

I didn't hear from her again until one day when I was sitting alone in the lobby of a local hotel awaiting the arrival of out-of-town friends. Mary came walking through on the way to the restaurant. She saw me and came over to tell me we had a long-term cure on our hands. It had been eight years since she'd stopped treatment. She was happy, well, successful in relationships, never again suicidal, never again had abused alcohol or drugs. I was both happy and dumbfounded. I pleaded with Mary to tell me, in long-term hindsight, what had been different in her treatment with me than with her previous therapists. I confessed I had been, was still, an inexperienced therapist who didn't know what he was doing except trying to help his patients with their goals and to figure out how he could be a more effective doctor. I knew I had no special skills and wasn't grandiose enough to think there was anything unique about what I do.

It was then that Mary uttered a simple statement—the one that focused my thinking for the rest of my career and since. She said, "All those other doctors treated me as if I'd be well when they fixed me. You treated me as if there were nothing wrong, and I'd be OK as soon as I knew that."

When one understands how ┃ *the originally implanted ideas* ┃ *perverted emotions,*
then entirely new concepts about behavior and feelings—based on adult realities, not infantile
misconceptions—offer a new potential for personal happiness and social harmony.

PART TWO

The World Turned Upside Down

Splitting Hairs and Popsicle Sticks and Cholera

KAY ENJOYED A BIT of irony, and some of my twisted thinking amused her to the point that she readily accepted ideas that were sometimes presented bizarrely and with a bit of humor, to say the least. I'm taking liberties with definitions and am saying things that are outrageous if taken out of context. I will try to explain what it is I mean with these absurdities. When I would do this with Kay, I would have the time to explain exactly what I meant, and I would look at the comprehension or lack thereof written on her face. I could be drawn and quartered for many of the statements herein unless one understands the specifics of what is intended. We're going to split hairs, microscopically redefine terms, and make use of popsicle sticks as polarities to figure out what I am trying to say.

I'm not writing anything I don't mean and believe. The purpose of my shenanigans will not be to rile or shock a reader; perhaps it will be to get the attention of my hoped for audience. I am going to say some things to purposely confuse the reader because I have found when the explanations unwind there is an imprint on the mind that makes these useful tools for achieving increased happiness. "Orange Is the New Black" is ludicrous and bad advice if I'm shopping for a tuxedo, but it's a catchy title, and if you understand the iconic stature of the little black dress, you will never forget what color is often found on prison garb. My point is you'll remember this if you see someone in an orange jumpsuit hitchhiking near Folsom as you're driving through California.

All of this is done in complete seriousness. Patients were trusting me with their careers, their lives, the upbringing of their children, and their personal relationships with mates. They were paying me with what to a lot of them was serious money. I would never take that lightly, even if I were to put an idea into a silly or catchy phrase to make it noted and remembered. I equally value your time in reading this book, and even when being silly or sarcastic or salacious, I am being deadly sober.

In usual language, "I don't want to go," is said when one means, "I want to not go." So, before we start, let's understand this: I don't want to go means I do not have a desire (to go). I want to not go means I do have a desire (to not go). I'm digressing to this because in the rest of this book I'm going to be making a lot of statements that have to be understood with this exactness. I'll make a point of clarifying, but I'm warning you to not be dismayed at what might seem as absurdities in some of my distinctions.

I am going to make a big deal of the difference between being responsible for something terrible and being to blame for something terrible. I will argue the R word and the B word are entirely different in connotation. This seems inane until one understands the tremendous power of microscopic differences in becoming a happier person. I will definitely be splitting hairs, for which I do not offer an apology.

There are two glasses of water on the table. Both appear exactly the same from every observation—equally clear, cool, and identical in taste. One will kill you, and the other will refresh you. The difference is microscopic. One contains cholera, and the other does not. Further, both contain bacteria; it will take an expert at a microscope to know one from the other. When I split hairs about blame versus responsibility, sorrow versus sadness, and excuse versus cause, I do so with purpose. Part of what it takes to make a person unhappy or happy is at stake. With that glass of water and those bacteria, the difference is only life or death.

I wish to call attention to the unconscious polarities that exist in our minds. It's as if we had an infinite supply of popsicle sticks each labeled with opposite nouns or adjectives on the two ends, which we unthinkingly align. The north end of one stick would line up with the good end of another (unless we were Australian) and the big end of a third. This is context specific, of course. Black would be north if we were thinking of finances, south if we were white racists; bigger would be south if talking about a waistline, north if talking about a penis. I want to reinforce that when I mention the word positive it should not be assumed to be good. Good should not be assumed to be desirable. Pain should not be assumed to be undesirable. Green does not necessarily mean go. I'm cautioning against automatically aligning polarities.

I make much use of seeing some sticks as assets and others as debits, both poles being accepted. If the two ends of a stick are labeled with symptoms, the stick is sick. If the two ends of a stick are labeled with emotions, the stick is healthy. Sadness and joy are equally healthy. Shame and pride are equally unhealthy. So, sadness would line up with shame, and pride would line up with joy, but sadness is not on the same unhealthy stick as shame, and pride is not on the same healthy stick as joy.

Often in psychotherapy–to the amazement of new therapists–a patient's behavior or symptoms might be interpreted many times during many sessions, and the patient will agree with the interpretation each time. Then, in a session weeks or months later, the patient will come in excited with some self-revelation discovered during the previous week. It will be exactly the same interpretation that had been voiced over and over for weeks and which the patient had enthusiastically accepted. But that didn't mean they got it. They got it during the week prior to the Aha! session.

To try to facilitate that breakthrough, the psychiatrist may rightfully attempt to say the same thing repeatedly in as many different ways as possible. You will find me writing the same idea that I've related before, sometimes immediately before, and you may grouse about my repetitive style. But each telling will be an attempt to show some facet from a varying angle. I also find that basic principles have numerous applications. I think iterating the basic with each new application makes the basic clear.

9

There Is No Such Thing as Bad

THE FEAR OF BEING wrong or the fiction that others are wrong is a major part of anxiety, depression, worry, guilt, shame, blame, and unfortunate behaviors. Every time a therapist is able to help a patient with such a symptom, they do so by lessening the patient's abasement of self, which the patient has based on some variant of the idea of wrong or bad. This is true for any style of psychotherapy, be it psychoanalytic, hypnotic, gestalt, cognitive, or supportive. It is also true of religion and of effervescent self-helpers. But they all fail to convey that bad does not exist.

Here's an analogy: Samuel is going through life terrified of being gored by a unicorn. He lives in a milieu in which there are horses everywhere, and every time he sees any part of a horse or hears hoof beats or a whinny, his life is disrupted by fear of unicorns. He is ashamed of being a coward, won't leave his house, accuses those without this fear of being ignorant or careless, can't make a living, and doesn't sleep on many nights. Therapists try to convince Sam he should not be ashamed of his fear, try to get him to go out in spite of his fear, and try to decondition his fear. They give him pills to quiet his racing heart and help him sleep. They psychoanalyze the origins of his fear. They testify in court that he shouldn't be responsible for his behavior because he is so afraid. But no one has ever told Sam there is no such thing as a unicorn—in spite of the pictures of them in books and the place they hold in myth.

A lot of people in this milieu get along just fine even though they also would not like to be run through by a unicorn. They check and see that every horse has no horn. They might even find it irrelevant whether or not there is such an animal. Some of them might believe such beasts do exist; others don't, but they all act as if they believe in unicorns because those who do not are branded by their society as a threat. The culture of my patient, Sam, supports his belief in unicorns but tries to diminish his fear. Those ignorants could benefit from any type of therapy and be helped to lead a less disturbed life with their belief in unicorns intact. But what a marvelous change could come over them and such a population of sufferers if they could understand unicorns are a fiction just like Santa Claus and the Tooth Fairy! If they could be helped to see those animals just don't exist, it would be the very best kind of therapy for that symptom.

There is an abyss of difference between being taught by self-helpers, preachers, teachers, psychiatrists, parents, and peers that the unicorns won't get you, that they will protect your from the unicorns, that you can resist the unicorns, etc. versus really understanding unicorns don't exist. Understanding that right/wrong and good/bad don't exist has the same benefit.

Learning that right/wrong and good/bad don't exist is what happens when one is Born Again. Knowing that is getting the right grip on the racket. It does not make everything OK, but it's what one needs to do to start over in the quest for happiness.

I'm arguing our lives are happier if we stop seeing ourselves, those with whom we interact, and those who appear on our ballots as bad or good. One cannot make this statement without having to logically deal with the ultimate extreme. I've never had this conversation—the one in which I pontificate that no one is bad—without a listener bringing up Hitler. Never. I really don't believe this horrid character was made awful by badness. He was made horrid by variant neurology, brain chemistry, sociological and psychological factors not understood, and his psychosis, which popped up in seriously the wrong place at the wrong time. I'd have slain him if I had been in the right place at the right time and could have predicted his future, not because he was bad but to save the lives of millions of victims. What was said about Eve before she met the snake would apply equally to Hitler before his mind was deformed in some way science has yet to explain, before his penis was maimed by the goat, and before his character was perverted, or if you prefer, before he was possessed by a devil. I do believe evil exists, and he was evil—meaning what he was and did was what we sincerely didn't want.

There is no goodness or badness in anyone. When we realize this about our children, our pets, our friends, our mates, our fuck buddies, and ourselves, we take one giant step toward being happier people.

A great benefit to one's happiness and mental health comes from practicing these ideas as if they are true, whether or not they are, but that behavior is more easily accomplished if one can accept what I said about right and wrong back in chapter 6.

When someone insults me and I act as if they are telling me something interesting about themselves, I will be a happier person (BA) than if I behave in the normal way of feeling shame or guilt (BS) or, equally normally, strike back to protect myself from shame or guilt (SOB).

If I end up in a dangerous back alley, I'll be a healthier person if I act as if I'd better learn quickly, act in a manner that will protect myself, get out of there, and don't come back through this part of the neighborhood again, but I do not do the normal thing of berating myself for not knowing better than I did. This is true whether I stumbled into the alley while lost or had dared to take it as a shortcut, and this is true whether I leave the alley wiser or end up robbed and bleeding into the cracks of the pavement.

Good and bad are like the gods. To the extent we think we understand something, we call it science; if we don't, we call it God. If we think we know why a serial killer murders, we call it sociopathy, perversion, or psychosis, and we try to understand the permutations of these concepts and update them as we learn more. If we don't have a clue and don't care that we don't think, we just say they are bad.

There are situations in life that require more advanced judgment than what has been mastered at any given instant—when one's maturity level is less than the occasion demands. In every moment of one's life, one has a capacity to grow further in the appreciation of the consequences of actions. By that standard, everything I ever did is less mentally advanced than what I might do now. This fact has nothing to do with badness.

If I understand why my child disobeyed me, played with matches, and burned down the house, I may wish he'd had better judgment a moment earlier than he did, but if I don't understand, then he is just bad. But, wait, I just used the word disobeyed. Well, readers, disobeying is good sometimes and bad sometimes (meaning only that we do or don't like the outcome), and the child uses the most maturity he has at any given moment. We understand children, up to the age of about ninety-three, have conflicts about rebellion, exercising their power, wanting to be sexually attractive, and on and on. Their level of judgment will increase until they lose their minds or die. That is not bad or good. Abraham Lincoln disobeyed the U. S. Constitution.

Each person is doing the best they can at the instant they act. I can always do better in the next instant—that's what keeps me motivated for a more joyful life, but I can't be better in the current instant than I am. To ask me to do so would be to ask me to have better wisdom, maturity, sense, intelligence, coordination, etc. than I have got. It's not possible at any instant to have better wisdom, maturity, sense, intelligence, coordination, etc. than one does have at that instant. And I don't believe in better. As you now know, it really means only more to my liking.

When I was a tall, skinny youth, being muscular and big was the sexy in-style. About the time I developed a furry chest, being smooth and blond was the ideal. For these and other reasons I saw myself as being unattractive. Not only that, I also saw being unattractive as worse than awful and became shameful about my own body. What a crock. I had the body of a slim, Italian model in the era when big and burly was better. Later styles changed, and I became beautiful? Because fashion had changed? I do admit if a child grows up with his style being the in-style, he has a great head start in the area of self-esteem. But with further exploration the value of self-esteem itself evaporates.

I went through much of my life feeling I was defective in not being adequately sexy. Now I understand that I was a perfect, skinny nerd. A skinny nerd who has confidence and knows what he is is sexy! I thought my cock was too small. Now I know it was perfectly normal or tiny or large or humongous or little and the whole question should have been what did I want to do with it. Was Napoleon too short? Some historians think the world might have been spared a lot of bloodshed had he been tall. I say his century might have been calmer had he internalized being OK the way he was.

A lefty is perfect while having an uncoordinated right. A homosexual is as perfect in loving and mating as is someone attracted to the opposite sex. A nerd is as perfect as is the jock. The woman who wants to ride horses, the man who wants to grow beans, the Romeo who happens to be five foot four and the child who is tone deaf are all perfect examples of what they are. We don't know what causes autism, but when we learn we will be able to see ourselves as no better than they in the same sense that our whole leg was not superior to the one with the bone poking out through the Bogners. And what if a bone breaks because it has osteogenesis imperfecta? That still doesn't mean that badness or need for shame is in that leg.

On several occasions I've constructed picture frames. Each time I've had a tricky task getting the four corners to fit as I have only two hands, and I never bought the proper clamps. I've often thought how much easier it would be if I had three hands. I have been angry when the project took forever or fell apart, but I've never felt shame or guilt that I didn't have three hands. That's the same as it is with our maturity, judgment, wisdom, ability to delay gratification, etc. I may wish I had more, perhaps a tragedy could have been avoided if I had had more, but I needn't have shame or guilt that I wasn't more advanced than I was at the point in time when the tragedy happened—or that I didn't have more hands. This is qualitatively true regardless of the quantity of the resultant grief.

I never bought useful clamps because each time I was about to make a frame I believed I would not be making any others, and the grief of only having two hands was less than the grief of the errand and the money it would have taken to go and buy the clamps. I was also not wrong in being unable to predict future craft projects.

If any desired result requires me to have three natural hands, or better wisdom, maturity, or judgment than I've got, then that result is going to cause sadness. If your life depends on me being taller than I am, having bluer eyes than I've got, being smarter than I am, being able to delay gratification better than I can, being more sexually secure than I am, being more rested than I am, or having a more stable blood sugar than I've got, you—no matter how much I love you—are going to die. I strive to grieve, grow, learn, cry, and change those things I can without feeling shame, blame, and guilt that I wasn't more than I was an instant earlier.

When I hear someone spouting, "You are perfect in every way," I tend to dismiss their drivel as new age, moonbeam, crystal-gazing crap. But I'm not seeing what I should be seeing when I think that way. I'm repeating the lie that they are wrong instead of grasping their optimism. If

I get out of my infantile rut, I may be able to see that the plants in my garden which I yank out because I don't want them there are just as perfect in themselves as are the plants I labor to put there. It's all a matter of which ones I like and which ones I don't like. Some plants that save lives when dosed properly for their medicinal value will kill children or dogs who gnaw on them. The idea of protecting ourselves from danger works for me, not the idea of bad or good. I may not need to protect myself from a flower child.

It seems to me in reflecting on the above ideas, it would be awfully self-righteous to assume I am not somehow bad if I have hurt you or have spilled the milk. In fact, it's the opposite because what I believe about myself I also believe about everyone else in the world.

I'm writing about how to be a happier person. When you thoughtlessly dent someone's car, you'll have a better day if you realize you just learned you will dent less cars in the future if you pay more attention than you thought you needed to pay than if you berate yourself for being _____ (insert here any synonym for bad or for something of which you'd be shamed). When your child disobeys, you'll be a happier parent if you realize it's a normal child who needs to learn something than if you think they are a bad child. When your puppy chews up your Ferragamos, anger is justified, blame is not—of yourself or the puppy; certainly the dog wasn't bad, and you weren't bad for hocking your children's future education for that pair of python loafers. Your everyday life will improve if you just get rid of bad, wrong, blame, and shame. This is true regardless of Stalin, Vlad, Idi Amin or any understanding of how my idea applies to them.

I think gravity is a good example of why the last paragraph is important. Knowing not to remain next to a brick wall during an earthquake does not require understanding gravity as it relates to the orbits of the planets. To make ourselves happier we need to understand how to apply the concept that we are not bad to ourselves and what we do every day even if we don't understand how it applies to Nero. But if there were to be a serious discussion about the nature of gravity, we'd have to know it works for Newton's apple and for Einstein's relativity. For a discussion of good and bad to be serious, it must apply to our daily drivel as well as deeds of barbaric beasts.

Witches were bad until we understood epilepsy and psychosis—and the manipulations of prosecutors seeking political power even in old Salem. Just as in the twentieth century lefties stopped being sinister when researchers came to understand lateralization of the brain, now in the twenty-first, there is neurochemistry research that seeks to separate conservatives from liberals, believers from doubters, queers from breeders, and slobs from neat freaks on the basis of previously unguessed neurology and chemistry. Some day, in my poor guess, we'll understand the difference between brutality, banality, and beauty and between narcissism, neighborliness, and nastiness, and it won't be on the basis of goodness or badness. I don't believe one must explain what happened to Pompeii on the basis of debauchery, and I don't believe the explanation of Rasputin or King Herod depends on sin.

"There is nothing either good or bad,
but thinking makes it so."

WILLIAM SHAKESPEARE

10

Anger Never Hurt Anyone

THIS SUBJECT EVOKES THE LOUDEST protests of any I broach, but it is a necessary part of being Born Again in the service of making for happier adults. I warn you to please have patience with me and to remember the glass full of perfectly fine water contaminated by lethal cholera bacilli. There's nothing wrong with the water, but the germs will kill you. Ever since we were first told not to be angry, or even were comforted in an attempt to allay anger—long before our current memory begins—anger has been mixed with shame or fear of anger just like the bacilli is mixed with the water. If we're all dying of cholera and I'm so absurd as to insist it's not the water, then I'm doing the same thing when I insist anger never hurt anyone. If I were an epidemiologist trying to save a city from cholera, I'd need to understand the difference between water and bacilli. If I'm trying to teach people how to be happier, I need for them to understand the healthiness of pure anger as separate from the deadly effects of being afraid of anger or even uncomfortable with it.

You and I were taught to somehow, consciously or unconsciously, abase ourselves whenever we were angry, and we could only lessen that abasement if we could find reason to blame another instead. Anything you see as being potentially untoward about anger, I would see as coming from that associated abasement, not from the anger itself.

Like a person suffering from cholera needs more hydration from uncontaminated water, not less water, so the person with anger problems needs to learn purer anger, not try to diminish their anger.

Anger is the good, positive, desired, expected, healthy, and safe emotion one experiences when one doesn't get what one wants. Anger contaminated with fear of anger causes murders, wars, battered spouses, abused children, smashed police cruisers, high blood pressure, and other mischief.

Whenever I've taught this, the patient has thought my insistence that this emotion is caused by merely not getting what one wants makes the subject out to be infantile, spoiled, or trivial. Bingo! That's my point—the ubiquity of this lethal falsity. The first time through that's exactly what we are taught. I agree one's behavior at not getting what one wants can be spoiled, spiteful, stupid, shitty, and dangerous, but the anger is not. It is the normal emotion. That's not explained to us—can't be explained to us—when we, as infants, are being conditioned against anger. We're simply told we're childish, churlish, or craven to be angry. No difference is made between being angry and acting angry. Acting angry is not caused by being angry; acting angry is caused by trying to not be angry. Lashing out, screaming, passive aggression, and cursing are attempts to make anger go away.

It's only in being Born Again that one learns the safety of having the pristine emotion without the dangerous defenses against it. When one doesn't get what one wants, one is angry. That anger can be denied, dismissed, disguised, or it can be so slight that it just isn't noticed, but it is there. If we see it as appropriate to the fact we didn't get what we wanted, we can go on from there with constructive planning about what to do. But if we suppose it is an unacceptable emotion unless someone is to blame for something, then we have a problem. If I can only be OK with myself for being angry if someone or something is to blame, then every time I don't get what I want I will want to blame something or punish someone. If I understand that anger is just the healthy emotion I'm supposed to have when I don't get what I want, then my psyche doesn't need to assault anyone.

We were all told, "Honey, don't be angry with Mommy; Mommy was just doing what she had to do to protect you." It was not noticed by Mommy, but she just made the child wrong for being angry. Later the kid is logically forced into the Shift of Blame. They're wrong to be angry unless–shift–Mommy is wrong to have done what she did. Think of the adults you know who just can't live with it unless they can right a wrong by punishing or at least blaming. Thankfully, they don't all go blow up a post office, but this is why the ones who do, do.

One would think that Mommy was just trying to get the infant to not be angry, not make the baby wrong for being angry. If there's nothing wrong with being angry, why was she trying to get the kid to not be angry? Initially she was just trying to soothe the child; she rocks and coos. Follow it, though, through a few stages of development. Soon an unequivocal directive arises to not show anger; to the receiver–to people in general–this message is taken to mean don't be angry. In the years of toddlerhood, a child will get a myriad of responses: you should not be angry, it's your own fault, the offender is not to blame, if you had only . . . , or a simple shut up.

Nothing in infancy teaches us to see violence or untoward behavior as being anything in itself. It is just seen as being what anger is. If we fear violence, then we fear anger. The concept of reveling in anger while doing nothing violent is a Born Again idea, an idea just not there in the original breeding.

I picture a nine-year-old child who smashes a model airplane they are building because they can't get a part to fit. The kid is not going to be supported that the anger is healthy. They are going to be told they should have been more patient or more, well, more something. They will learn to do it with more something next time, but it is not true that they should have been more anything this time, and though the destruction may be untoward, the anger is not.

Consider a little boy who is scratched by his cat. Likely responses from an attentive parent might include comforting the boy, blaming the cat, blaming the boy, or giving the kid some instruction on how to better relate to the cat. It is not likely that the child will be made to feel good about the fact he is angry. Many modern parents are encouraging their children to go ahead and be angry these days, but I've yet to encounter many who really believe that other than when the anger is justified. Believing anger to be natural and normal and healthful just because one didn't get what one wanted still seems to be cutting edge.

Anger is not subject to rational thought, even thought about whether or not one would really want what one did not get, and fear of anger is toxic even when applied to any minor degree of hurt. You might think gravity is an insignificant thing if it just pulls the quarter you're about to insert into a parking meter down into a sidewalk grate. But that same gravity is what destroys planets and stars in the cosmos, and it kills when an airplane falls out of the sky. Likewise, the fear of anger could cause one to think that they shouldn't get so upset over a trivial issue or it could cause another to murder because they just can't stand the emotion that has emerged.

When I would treat a patient who had just had a parent or child murdered, or someone who had suffered an accident that had killed their children, I was in no way trivializing their horror to see it as my job, sometimes over much time, to help them understand the rightness of their anger and grief as a separate emotional experience from shame, blame, guilt, or the need for revenge. The scene is qualitatively the same (though quantitatively, astronomically different) as when one is angry the coin went into the grate, but then the emotion is fouled by blame of one-self that one dropped the quarter unless one can blame another, as if for causing a distraction.

Thankfully, horrible events are rare, but common and everyday are the little applications of this fix that will increase the common and everyday happiness of those who understand the idea of being angry absent blaming anyone for anything.

I had a friend who once became so angry when a lifelong friend of his wouldn't agree about the size of an ancient doorway that they hadn't spoken in nine years. My ex-friend couldn't just be angry that the friend wouldn't agree and then drop it. He had to see something trivial as being significant in order to justify his anger. It wasn't how wrong was the other person, it was how much my friend was afraid to be angry. Of course, the reason he was so angry with his friend was that the friend wouldn't validate him as being right. Then he had to make the friend wrong and do something to punish the wrong—in this case shun his friend.

Normal children grow up to become the people who drive to a store at five fifteen only to find it closed at five o'clock and say some version of "I should have known," or "I should have called to check on their hours." Or, more likely, they may blame the store for its hours of operation. It's not likely they will just be angry they didn't get what they wanted. They may decide they'll never patronize that store again or, maybe, won't go to any store without calling to check the hours of operation first. They might start shopping only at a major mall. They might see this as happening so rarely that nothing needs be done. There needs be a decision of what they want to do now about what they learned, but there does not need to be a sense that they, or another, were wrong to have not done so before they learned. Absent a fear they were wrong, maybe nothing needs to be done except to come back later.

I got a comeuppance on my own inability to practice what I preach when I was walking to my gym on the morning on which I wrote this paragraph. I passed a neighbor whom I quite like, respect, and enjoy greeting. I thought back to the first time I had met this neighbor and how long it had taken (time I had wasted) to see her as someone I'd befriend. It happened that I had been having a quiet party at a time when I felt no one could reasonably take umbrage over what little sounds were coming out of my house. This neighbor showed up at my front door to request, politely, that we make less noise. From the perspective of this morning, I can look back and see how I failed to just be an ounce angry at the ounce of intrusion. I had to blame myself for being a bad neighbor unless I justified my behavior and saw the woman at the door as unreasonable and inappropriately controlling. Had I only been angry over her asking for quiet when I wanted to make noise and had done what I wanted to do about that, I would have said, "Rats!" and lowered the volume, maybe grumbled a bit, and then would have sooner been able to enjoy the things which I later came to enjoy about her. This seems so tiny that I would criticize myself for wasting the ink to tell the story except that it is a huge exaggeration of this same point that leads some to take a gun to the neighbor.

The racism that can lead to a hate crime murder is nothing more than an obscenely blown up version of this same thing: I'm angry about facing someone or some group that makes me uncomfortable on the basis of some prior teaching or experience. I defend against any internal suggestion I could be less than ideal, therefore the other is unacceptable, and I'm unable to face myself unless I can do something to cleanse my environment of this vermin—or punish them. It's been long understood that racism, homophobia, religious intolerance, along with simple jealousy come from internalized shame over feared inadequacy, but I want to make a point here of what is usually not mentioned—that the doing of any offense from a hate crime down to a simple insult comes from the inability of the perpetrator to be at ease with his anger at the loathed scapegoat of his own frozen, impotent confidence.

Everyone has heard that depression is anger turned inwards. As my psyche was polluted with BS before I could learn to speak and later, I learned the SOB exception that it wasn't my fault if it was your fault. I learned to debase myself unless I could blame you when I wasn't getting what I wanted. If I blamed, I could allow myself to be angry at you; otherwise, I "turned the anger inward" and became depressed (self-blame). As an example: if you dis me, then I must be an ass or else you're a bastard. Maybe both. But one is on the tipping balance of I'm crummy or else you're crummy or maybe were both crummy. In the ultimate, psychotic manifestation of the myth, I must suicide if I can't murder—it's (the anger) turned inward if it's not turned outward. Of course, that horror only happens occasionally, thankfully, but understanding all of this must be as basic as ABC for a psychiatrist. We all go through the BS or Shift of Blame in much smaller ways daily, and it is always a source for unhappiness.

If one does not believe the BS, anger doesn't need to be turned anywhere. There is no blame of oneself or of any other. To be Born Again is to be at peace with having the appropriate emotion (anger) instead of blaming oneself or another when something is amiss.

When one finds one's spouse in bed with one's best friend, the simplest response for a Born Again adult is to be angry, very angry, if that's not what they wanted. One might be angry about this forever. Now, the behavior called for is to either jump into a three-way or else find something else to do—at that moment or with one's life or about choosing new friends and a new spouse. But there is no reason based on anger to do anything.

I know this may be impossible to comprehend at the moment it happens. It might be very hard not to feel less a man because my friend and my wife would do this to me. It's my own fault. Or else (SOB) I would prove I am a man by killing them—after all, they are just trash. At this point it's just not possible to not take it personally. But we'll get to that in future chapters.

When I would talk to a patient about just accepting the anger as the appropriate emotion, the patient would always say, "But then, how does one get over the anger?" I'd respond with, "Well, when you are happy about something, how do you get over the happy?" Happy is what you are supposed to feel when you get what you want; anger is what you are supposed to feel when you don't get what you want. There is no getting over either; they just take their allotted space in your mind. If I think about the time a toy broke when I dropped it as a child, I'm still angry it wasn't stronger, but I haven't thought about it in sixty-eight years. If I think of how excited I was when I got my first toy train, I'm happy, but I haven't thought of it in sixty-seven years. The trick is to get over the "taking it personally" when I'm angry. It does not mean there was anything wrong with me, and it doesn't mean I should have had some satisfaction by getting even with anyone. Now, of course, there are things in my past about which the anger or the happiness was such that I do still think of it every day. But I'm at peace with the emotion, and I don't need to get over it. That helps it go to a back burner. Understanding and accepting the true emotion is the closure.

Understanding the SOB explains why those victimized by a murderer need to see the offender executed to have closure. They can't live in peace with their anger until they see the punishment. They still believe they are somehow impotent, without value, vulnerable, and they are at terrible internal unrest until they see the Shift of Blame result in the debasement, conviction, agony, and death of the perpetrator. When a white cop kills a black person and gets away with it, the news features a relative of the victim proclaiming it's as if they don't matter. They are right in their protest, and I protest with them. But they do matter, and they matter just as much whatever may be done with the cop or whatever was the precipitant for the homicide.

At the other end of the scale is the kid in school who is taken advantage of or made fun of and suffers loss of self-esteem until they "get even."

Turning the other cheek is good advice to tell a congregation whom you want to lead to God. On an individual basis I think it's only using latent guilt over anger to batter the offended into inaction. Without understanding the BS and the SOB, the victim just represses more anger. This works pretty well. There are voters who will vote against their best interests if the party leaders can convince them God wants them to, so it seems equally possible that the preacher man can get his flock to sit and smolder on their anger if they are told that God wants them to. I don't think this adds to happiness unless one is happy when thinking their suffering is a way into heaven. On the other hand, when one does not blame and understands that their anger, no matter how intense, does not need to be assuaged, one is wiser at deciding what to do about having been struck in the face. Maybe the bully needs to be ignored, maybe beaten up, maybe sued in court, or maybe castrated and forced to eat his testicles. (Gee isn't it fun when one doesn't fear one's fantasies?) But the point is to do what needs to be done about the situation—not about the anger. Nothing needs to be done about the anger.

One is a lot happier to just learn shit happens. Eighty-two percent of life is good, 15 percent is bleh, and 3 percent is awful. We must grow to be at peace with being happy 82 percent of the time, bored 15 percent of the time, and angry 3 percent of the time–forever. There is no god who doesn't love you. It doesn't mean you were deficient. But if the 15 percent or the 3 percent causes frustration instead of simple anger, then that 18 percent metastasizes and invades the 82 percent to the point where it can ruin one's life.

It's no different if a loved one is murdered, if the boss is unfair, or if your spouse cheats with your best friend. Life is a bitch and then you die. The only way to tolerate this reality is to learn how to enjoy the 82 percent while still hating the part that isn't the way that you want.

People would say to me, "But it seems to me my life is bad 82 percent of the time." My counter would be it seems that way because everything that makes you mad makes you think there is something wrong with you or else you must feel shame you didn't get even. The ones with the issues don't see that they are magnifying the issues to make everything be about themselves.

When you get a dent in your new car, all you see is the dent. One needs to concentrate on the fact that 99.99 percent of the car is fine and still be furious about the 0.01 percent. One will, instead, obsess on the dent because unconsciously they can't accept they will be angry at just not having what they want–a perfect car. So, they have to get depressed–hate themselves for being angry–or they have to make the fact the car has a dent be a big deal to justify their anger. Back to the actual percentage, I'd say if I can count to twenty-one on my body's appendages and have food, shelter, and clothing, then 82 percent of my life is good.

So here's my idea of anger management. I feel anger. I dwell on it. I sit down, put my head in my hands, squeeze a little, and remind myself I don't have what I want and am damn angry about it. I should be angry; I should be as angry as I can possibly make myself. I don't have to move, strike, fart, or make a comment. I'm just at peace with the fact that I'm angry. Next, what to do? Well, what behavior on my part will give me the short- and long-term consequences with which I wish to live, using good judgment while not having to assuage the anger? Unfaithful spouse: maybe honest communication, maybe a new spouse, maybe an open marriage–whatever. Boss being an asshole: maybe a confrontation, maybe a change in my need to please him, maybe a new job, maybe slashing his tires–whatever, with adult judgment, I choose to live with the consequences thereof.

My life will be unsatisfying if for everything that's wrong I feel I'm wrong unless I can fix it, unsatisfying if I feel everyone who offends me is evidence of my impotence if I can't correct or punish them, unsatisfying if it should be better than it is. But life is happy if I am simply angry at all the things I don't like and pay equal attention to being glad about everything I do like. I go after everything I want and make myself happy with those things I get. I'm angry I have to do without the rest, but I'm glad I'm angry about it, without blame and shame and without a sense life should be better.

Here's a very practical and trivial example of how this chapter makes me a happier person. I recently got my first puppy in forty-five years. I've had adult dogs since, which I had rescued. In taking on the eight-week old pup, I had unreal expectations on how housebreaking gets accomplished. I would get angry when I found piss or shit in the house but would heroically hide the anger from the pup and do as I'd learned I was supposed to do. After this went on for a longer period of time than I thought reasonable, I started to become discouraged. My dog trainer, Ryan Furlet, observed what I was doing and commented I was doing exactly the right thing, and when the dog got a little older the housebreaking would be successful. I didn't need to make myself or my pup wrong to explain my anger. Since that revelation, my anger at my dog doesn't bother me. Even while writing this chapter, I still wasn't seeing that my own anger was fine and the puppy was fine until Ryan commented. When I applied to myself and my dog what I've been applying to paper, the sense of being OK resolved the stress. In a less aware individual, such stress could have led to the puppy being brutalized, but it was of that intensity because I was, unseeingly, blaming myself that the dog hadn't already learned.

A usual technique for a psychiatrist to use when dealing with a patient's discouragement or depression is simply to get the patient to understand he is angry and hating himself for being angry. Just the verbalization of permission for the patient to be angry lifts the depression some-what. Now, a therapist doesn't use words that aren't obvious to the situation if he wants to be useful to the patient, and he doesn't overanalyze. It seems paradoxical, but an everyday occurrence in psychotherapy happens when a patient comes in depressed or discouraged and will tell the psychiatrist what ill is happening. The therapist will say, "Oh, that is terrible!" and the patient will say, "Oh, thank you, doctor; you've made me feel so much better." Again without scientific data, I believe uncovering unconscious anger and permitting a patient to safely see that anger is the single most used element in the practice of psychotherapy.

In a seminar I was conducting, a woman wiser than I disagreed with me in my basic premise.

I was thinking of violence when I was claiming anger never hurt anyone. Laura (you met her back in chapter 2) reminded me, correctly, I had earlier made a big point of how the slightest emotion could change one's physiology. How could I say this could not hurt someone? Could not one have a heart attack triggered by a change in blood pressure? Could not anger without fear of the anger cause a change even if it were not as profound as that caused by anger with fear of anger? I readily agreed with Laura. She was correct; I was in error. In such a case anger could be dangerous—about as dangerous as winning the lottery.

Back in chapter 5, I made a point that conflicts about emotions cause symptoms, conflicted emotions do not. The great majority of symptoms that patients bring to therapists result from the conflict about an emotion causing the patient to be unaware and defensive about the emotion. This is why patients will come in befuddled about symptoms for which they can see no reason. If one is aware of, and OK with, loving and hating the same person, symptoms will not arise, but there will be a problem if hatred makes one unaware of one's love or if love makes one unaware of the hate. The problem is not one of love and hate; the problem is lack of awareness of one half of the conflict. Much more will be made of this shortly.

Since my midthirties I have at times developed hives on my body seemingly for no reason; they may last for hours and then just disappear. The no reason part of that sentence passed sometime before I was forty. I learned my body will do something with what is probably histamine if I am angry and do not know I am angry. Friends who know me well will ask me at times why I am angry. I will protest that I am not angry; I'm aware of no reason to be angry. They will then point out the emergence of my hives. I have learned to actually make the hives dissipate just by forcing my mind to get as angry as I can make it be. I don't even have to be aware of what I am angry about. I can actually make the hives go by faking anger, if I can really get into it.

To colorfully illustrate my point about the conflict over the emotion causing symptoms when conflicted emotions do not, I will share with you that on rare occasions I've developed these hives while having sex. For a time, I just broadened my belief about what was causing them to include sexual excitement, but I came to see this was wrong. The hives during sex would occur when I was so sexually hyped as to be unaware of being angry about having to be quiet because of an unfortunate location, because my partner was taking too long, or because of some other puzzle that might be inappropriate for me to share. We come across case histories daily of sexual dysfunction being caused by a conflict, but this was not sexual dysfunction; it was hives developing in the course of sexual function which was just splendid. What was said in the above paragraph worked in this paragraph as well. By concentrating on the object of the sexual excitement at the same time as allowing the anger at the imposition to become conscious, I would become a hive-free, happy fucker.

At a medical conference in New York City I had the chance to chat about this phenomenon with a doctor who was both an internist and a psychiatrist and who specialized in the narrow field of the interaction between mind and hormones. He told me there are many such stories for which no explanation has ever been proven—the research has not been done—but reminded me that tranquilizers have antihistamine action and antihistamines have tranquilizing effects.

11

Shame on You for Feeling Guilty!

I AM HAVING TROUBLE starting this chapter because I'm about to violate one of the most sacrosanct rules for any medical doctor when talking with a patient: "Never say *Never*; Never say *Always*."

Shame, blame, and guilt are NEVER appropriate. Punishment is ALWAYS a crime.

One can't really teach happiness without accepting this premise. Here's another place we part company with the tennis buddy who yells, "Hit it," and the motivational speaker who makes their money hyping up the masses.

At this point most everyone objects with, "But if we don't feel shame or guilt, what will keep us from becoming bad people?" We'll get to that. At this point let's just say shame and guilt cause us to not reach our full potential to become responsible, happy, loving, sharing, caring persons. They make our problems worse than they already were. Shame and guilt kill.

They kill the joy of life with everything they touch; they are a central element in most suicides and many murders. They cause some sufferers to stop living decades before they die. One can't really teach happiness until one learns how to lyse these emotions. Religions push a fictitious patch for the falsehood. Positive thinkers are distractions; addictions numb the suffering.

The fix for the calamities caused by these pitfalls is something I've not yet been able to use 100 percent of the time myself—as you'll see in a humorous situation a few paragraphs below. But I do know what it is; I can teach it; I can apply it to myself most of the time, and I applied it gently to sufferers who came to me suicidal, depressed to the point of total disability, and miserable. To live without joy for years is a tragedy as it is to shorten one's life by means of suicide.

On a much less dire note, look at yourself and your friends and ask how much happier you would be if you didn't know guilt or shame.

Harold was a patient with bipolar disorder who came to treatment when, in a normal state of mood, he realized he was in need of help. He had gone through a serious episode of depression about five years before following the loss of a job, and he and his wife had struggled to support their children in his period of recovery. About three years later he developed an episode of mania in which he left his supportive wife and spent everything he had earned back after the depression. He later came to see me broke and alone. With physical manifestations of shame and guilt he blurted out to me, "I can't believe I was so stupid." We had already established enough rapport that he was able to feel some relief when I told him, "Well, back then you really were that stupid, so stop blaming yourself."

One of the most difficult and important ideas for a person to grasp when being Born Again is the concept that they are to blame for nothing. This thought is so at variance with what we learned back in the Bullshit period that we just have to shut up and listen until the popsicle sticks, microscope, and hair splitting are understood. As we will see in chapter 24, we are responsible for everything. This is not in conflict with the idea of being to blame for nothing.

I do not feel blame over not being able to handle a tumbler of milk at age two as well as I could at age three. At three I couldn't do it as well as at five. In my eighth decade, I still can't handle one perfectly. Recently, in a fine restaurant, I toppled my beer into the lap of a lovely lady sitting opposite me whom I would never want to embarrass or inconvenience. When I did, I had a hard time trying to remember what I teach in order to not blame myself, as I was bred to blame myself when I spilled anytime after preschool. The fact I will spill things, break things, and bump into things for my entire life is not a cause for shame or blame or guilt. It may be the reason for which I end up paying dry cleaning bills of dinner companions, apologize a lot, or need to find new friends frequently.

Likewise, I need not blame myself when I acted on Tuesday without the knowledge Wednesday would bring. One need not blame oneself for not using the knowledge that came at 3:38:00 at 3:37:50 when making a certain comment at work and learning ten seconds later the boss was standing within earshot.

I continue to work at improving my nimbleness at the dining table, as I continue to work on not letting slip out statements that would compromise me were certain persons to overhear them, but I need not blame myself that at those moments I did the actions I did when I was not as tuned in to the extra need for care as I was a second later.

Remember Mazda therapy. I must Grieve the unpleasantness then Learn and Change the behavior. This I can do more efficiently if I don't blame myself. Blame does to the mind's eye what a cataract does to the anatomical eye.

Ewan came to my office seeking help; I don't remember why. It happened to come out, incidentally, that he had occasions of not being able to have an erection when masturbating. He, in locker room talk among the jocks in high school, had been instilled with the idea that wanking was something studs only did when they couldn't find a woman! Thus, one who was proud of his prowess with pussy would never admit to jacking off—oh, the shame! Thank the gods, that went out with the Eisenhower era.

One day Ewan told me of an experience in which he was very disgusted with himself. He had been in the Laguna Hills Mall where a Sears store was about a two-minute walk from a J.C. Penney. He had seen a power tool he wanted on sale at Sears and thought he should check the price for something similar at Penney's before he bought it. He didn't and just bought it at Sears. That night he saw in his newspaper a J.C. Penney ad for the same item, which was on sale for eighteen dollars less than he had paid at Sears. He said to me, "Damn me, I should have checked the price at Penney's before I bought it. I knew I should have done that, and I didn't." He rejected my argument that he had done the best he knew how to do at the time. He knew he had known at the time he should have checked the price at JCP. He had been raised to feel guilt if he wasted money by his parents who had left their adolescence during the Great Depression.

I asked him to take out his psycho-microscope and look back at the minute he made the decision to impulse buy at Sears. His wife was waiting in the car, he badly needed to piss, and he was tired. He quickly came to see he would have checked the price at Penney's if he had not been hurrying for his wife, had not had a full bladder, and had not been that tired. Given he was, he did make the best decision he could make. The psycho-microscope revealed something more. If those three circumstances had changed, he still might not have checked the price at Penney's because there was maybe a 10 percent chance it would be cheaper there. If it were cheaper, there was a 80 percent chance it would not be more than five dollars cheaper, he guessed. Under those circumstances he might make the choice, consciously or not, it wasn't worth the trip down the mall for a 2 percent chance of saving more than five dollars and a 90 percent chance of saving nothing at all. There clearly was no blame and no reason for him to castigate himself however he chose to address those odds. There was only reason for eighteen dollars worth of grief.

Does one learning to not shame oneself if something is not as it could be translate into less stroking dissatisfaction? I don't know, but that's the way it often works, and Ewan did harbor those absurd, childish messages that men who are desirable enough to have a woman don't masturbate. We don't have a double-blind study, so I can't say. Erections can be notoriously fragile in some people who are harboring conflicts over shame.

What about when I do something for which there is a huge consequence? The most grievous case I ever attended was the worst that can be. A woman came to see me after she had caused an accident, through inattention, which killed all her children. In another case a father had actually murdered his son in his childhood. There were others of almost the same seriousness.

The severity of the grief does not change the nature of the logic. The more grievous the event, the more grievous is the emotion and the more grievous is the outcome caused by fear of the emotion. But the nature of the fact that I cannot use at any given instant the sanity, the compassion, the wisdom, the knowledge, or the common sense of the next instant is still the way it is. This is not blamable. One is responsible; one is not to blame.

Years ago, David Jr. arranged for two of his friends to stay in my home for a few days when they came from New York to visit Laguna Beach. I had met them previously, liked them, and was glad to have them as houseguests. While they were here, I loaned them my car for a day to visit San Diego. While in the Dirty Waffle, they spent the day with a friend whom they let

90

drive the car because the friend knew the area and they did not. The friend backed my car into another resulting in an insurance claim for the other car and some damage to mine. At first I felt resentful because I told myself I was willing to take responsibility for my decision to entrust the car to the wisdom and driving abilities of the friends, but not to unknown friends of the friends.

Then it hit me: yes, I must take responsibility for having loaned my car to my son's friends to do with as their judgment dictated. I had trusted them to make decisions with regard to the car that day—how fast to drive, where to park, to curb the wheels on a hill, etc. The decision to let the friend who knew the area drive the car was a judgment of theirs, and I had to take responsibility for the fact I trusted the car to their judgment. I did not blame myself that I had done this. I did not blame the friends for letting their friend drive. I did not blame the friend of the friends for backing into another car. All of us had made our decisions the best we knew to make them. We each were responsible for our own actions, and we each would live with the consequences of our decisions. The cost, dent, insurance issues, and wisdom gained, were not that painful. Those were the only issues. Had the event been tragic, the amount of grief would have changed, but the blamelessness would have been the same. The blame and distrust that could have been in any degree of awfulness would have poisoned and resulted in unhappiness. It was in our best interest to take responsibility without blame. It became of such minor importance that I never mentioned it to Dave and didn't realize I had not. His friends made reference of the accident to him months later, and all were amazed I hadn't. Why is this story in a chapter on guilt? Back to the teeter-totter. If I don't believe the BS, I won't be susceptible to feeling guilt that I was somehow remiss in how I loaned the car, and then there is just no need to do the SOB thing (blame another).

One could say it is unwise to ever loan a car. That is also irrelevant. Just like Ewan who wanted to buy the saw and go piss before he retrieved his wife without going to Penney's, there are always reasons for doing what we do, and—even though those reasons may ride well below our threshold of observation—we always do what we actually want to do. This is not blamable. It is just the way it is.

If the Indian subcontinent bumped into Central Asia with less force, the Himalayas wouldn't be as tall as they are. That is not good, bad, right, or wrong. It's just the way it is. We are creatures with reason and land masses are not. That doesn't give us any ability to know to do differently at any given instant than we do. It would be just as impossible as it would be for rocks to think.

It is true that I also believe Bonnie and Clyde and George (W. Bush) were doing the best they knew. There is a lot of explaining to do to make sense of that; nevertheless, if I treat my children, my spouse, my associates, my enemies, and myself without blame, I will be a happier person.

Recently I was away from my pants for a few moments while engaged in a homoerotic orgy in Las Vegas when some lowlife stole my new iPhone from my front jeans pocket. I had a strange reaction, the exploration of which taught me even more about blame/guilt and how it was that—even while I teach this stuff—I couldn't practice what I preach. When I found the pocket empty, I had first a feeling of immediate panic, then a sick feeling, then fear, then anger. The whole event ended up causing me insomnia and a headache that lasted for ten days. I want to do a walk-through of my emotions to illustrate the role blame plays in our emotions—even when we don't believe in blame—and to illustrate the less-than-conscious nature of our emotions and, separately, that we never grow up; we never get it entirely or immediately right.

For the first couple of days after the event, I knew I was blaming myself because of the presence of the angst. Without the blame there would be anger, but not the degree of discomfort I was feeling and knew to be illogical. For over a day I struggled with the idea I was blaming myself for having abandoned my pants for those few moments when the phone was stolen. I couldn't embrace that idea, though, because at the time it had happened I had made a conscious decision I was taking a risk. My best judgment had been the risk was so small as to be worth taking, and my life taking some risks is better in quality than would be my life if I were never to take any risk at all. The similar risks I have taken have been such that I have lost precious little, so well below the benefits I have received from taking those risks that I have been convinced my level of risk-taking was pretty appropriate. In fact, life might actually be happier for me if I loosened up a little and took more risks.

A friend went to the point most people would have sensed immediately. Was I blaming myself because I was at an orgy? I was pretty sure not. What I finally figured out, over a week later, was I had failed to outsmart the thief. I wasn't as smart as I thought I was. When I realized this, the angst pretty much went away. I'm not smarter than I am any more than I can use three hands to make a picture frame, and it just happened I ran into a thief who was better at what he does than I was at preventing what he does. I could accept that when it floated up to my consciousness. I had been aware I had chosen to take a risk of losing the iPhone and that I had been at a party of questionable acceptability to my friend, but not that I was faulting myself for not being smarter than the thief. After I thought that through, I was left with grief I didn't have my phone, not much else. I also learned from the experience and will, next time, leave my phone at home when I don't see a way to keep it directly on my body. Mazda therapy: G, L, C.

I can't tap the beat of a Sousa march, much less dance at a disco. If I were at a concert when everyone started clapping along with the music, I'd have to either skip it or visually cue my clapping to what I see the person sitting next to me doing. Barbara was trying to teach me to dance one night at the bar in the Hotel Laguna. In the middle of the floor as she was moving to the music she said, "Dave, just do what you feel." I retorted, "Barbara, if I just do what I feel I will sit down and cry."

Einstein was noted for not being a good father. Richard Nixon wasn't satisfied to be the most powerful person in the world and self-destructed in a grab for more power. Mrs. Malaprop's feet (both of them) kept going in her mouth. George W. Bush committed war crimes without any concept of history or geography or cultures or what the heck he was doing. All of the above are sad to differing degrees, none of them are blamable. I won't even mention Bill sticking what he did down Monica's whatever. Responsible, yes; blamable, no. They couldn't do their dance either.

No one can use better emotional bonding, musical talent, self-control, intellect, wisdom, intelligence, learning, or propriety than one's got at a given instant. If one learns, one can do differently in a future moment. I'd believe in awarding custody to someone else, throwing me off the dance floor, impeaching a President, defeating at the polls, sending a war criminal to prison, and putting a chastity device on Bill's penis, but I don't believe in blaming them. And I could hate them before I'd look down on them.

Mike was a stateside US Navy pilot who came to see me because of a persistent sexual problem. He had a history of being more than experienced with intimates, one-night stands, and prostitutes. He'd never had a problem with premature ejaculation or impotence until such developed as he was getting emotionally closer and closer to his live-in girlfriend, Jessica. He had no embarrassment talking about the problem with me, with Jessica, or even with his buddies. That's unusual for someone with sexual problems. However mysterious, it was not amusing and was becoming more persistent to a point that just sucked big time. There was nothing about this woman to account for any ambivalence related to her. She was willing, exciting, sexually arousing, and nonjudgmental. The place where they lived was conducive to whatever experiences they wanted. I explored every potential avenue I could imagine and came up with nothing. I pursued the possibility of a homosexual conflict unconsciously emerging. Physical examinations and lab tests were as useless as my attempts in finding any clue. There was no medical reason; he wasn't abusing drugs or alcohol. I knew not to give up because there had to be something; the symptoms were persistent, and to Top Gun Mike they were devastating. Really confusing was the fact that Mike seemed sexually secure and sophisticated in talking so openly about his problem.

Then one day, Mike started talking about Nicholas. There was affection and concern in his voice, which made me wonder again about the sub rosa possibility of some homosexual conflict. I thank the gods I kept my mouth shut as he kept talking. Nick was his closest friend; both were Navy pilots. Mike's caring for Nick was charming and admirable, revealing Mike to be a genuinely noble fellow. I asked for more detail about Nick. Nick was facing all one faces in his current assignment–Nam! Suddenly Mike made an association. Mike's waning sexual abilities with Jessica paralleled in time the growth of worrisome news from Nick about increasing dangers associated with Nick's missions. I was getting confused about what were the associations between his sexual disabilities and Nick's peril. Rather than specific probing, I just asked Mike to keep telling me more about Nick.

To this day, I do not believe there was any duplicity or lack of motivation to be honest on Mike's part. He genuinely wanted help with his inability to function and was as open as he'd been able to be since session number one. It unbelievably hadn't occurred to him, until this moment, to tell me Jessica was Nick's wife. He'd started out helping his buddy by giving Nick's wife a place to stay while Nick was deployed to hell.

Why is this story in the chapter about not guilting? Because I don't know a better example of how one can't use wisdom, insight, street smarts, or introspection any better than one can. I'm not referring to Mike's screwing his best friend's wife. I'm referring to his blindness at not making the connection. He was that blind; I won't blame him for that blindness. I'm also not going to blame myself that in earlier sessions I hadn't asked him if he was bonking his best mate's wife while he was worried about that best mate's life. I might have guessed such could be so mainstream as to not be noticed had I been working in England or Australia, but not in puritan America.

At about two o'clock on a Sunday morning, the sixteen year-old who later became this writer was returning home from a date and fell asleep at the wheel on the Santa Ana Freeway in a big curve where the I-5 crosses Lincoln Avenue. I awoke in terror on the center median, steered right, and stood on the brake pedal. All I could think of was to dodge other cars and get the damned Ford stopped as I end-for-ended and slipped off the edge of the road. I hit nothing and didn't hurt the car. On the shoulder I got the car turned around and re-entered the roadway toward home with my body shaking faster than the car was moving. I pulled off onto Harbor Boulevard and crawled home the rest of the way on surface streets. I'm telling you this story because the minute my car was off the freeway, I was certain I had imagined the whole thing. I drove on surface streets more because I was doubting my mind than my driving abilities. The next morning I awoke early remembering I'd had this troubling delusion the night before. I would have sworn under oath in a court of law the event had been imagined, had never happened. I got in the car and drove back to the spot to find fresh skid marks on the divider and roadway exactly where I had left them four hours before.

Eons later I saw a man killed at my left hand. My son John was with me and screamed. I am absolutely sure in the fraction of a second between seeing him killed and hearing the scream, I had no concern anything unusual had happened. It was the scream that shocked me into knowing what I had seen was real.

A similar lapse addled a murder investigation near Los Angeles some time later. A decayed corpse had been found in a forest, and the case was pretty much solved except for the fact that in the month in which the coroner had decided that the deceased had died the logical suspect had been in prison. The alibi was perfect, but it evaporated when a witness came forward who had found the body in the woods two months earlier than had been the estimate of the coroner—at a time when the suspect was free. During the suspect's trial the defense, of course, made a big deal of how this witness could have found a body and never reported it until the case erupted in the media shortly before the trial had begun.

The witness claimed to have had exactly the same experience as did I on the freeway and later when the man was killed at my side. The events had been so wildly outside of what we expected to experience that we truly believed we had imagined the whole thing. The later events in the press about the body being found had the same effect on the witness as finding the skid marks on the freeway or hearing John scream had on me.

If I don't blame Mike for his blindness to the link between his worrying about Nick and his inability to screw Jessica, and if I don't blame myself for my grasp on what I do and see, then where would I get off blaming Mr. Bush for his guile that ended up killing hundreds of thousands?

Sometimes denial may be the result of wishful thinking. Well, I can't use better judgment about my wishful thinking at any given instant than I can about my shock and awe.

I'm using the stories in this chapter to try to make my point that denial, uncontrolled urges, immaturity, lack of insight, bad judgment, sexual passion, fear of anger, the effects of BS and the SOB, etc. are such in cases we can analyze that we can be sure those things go on in everybody, every day. That's just the way it is. We all have to live with the consequences of our behavior and those consequences dealt to us by parents, cops, teachers, and the officers of the court who are all equally burned by those same lapses. At times all of the above may cause tragedies, but it is not blamable that no one is more anything than they are.

Whether you buy my suppositions or not, I'd challenge you to examine for yourself how you feel if you look at any disobedient kid and, instead of seeing him as blamable or worthy of punishment, you get it that he's running on a program you can't see or understand. Acknowledge that for whatever is the known or unknown reason, he's doing the best he knows how to do. Without blame, take it as a puzzle to figure out how you are going to protect yourself from him, him from himself, him from you and adopt the same attitude you'd have if you were struggling with sudoku. Imagine yourself an ER surgeon trying to figure out how to remove an arrow that entered a victim's open mouth and is protruding from the back of the neck (another military incident with which I once dealt) when you are imagining what should be done with a serial killer. If you'd want to challenge me by going back to Herr Hitler, I'd still rather look for a solution, as one would have to do if fighting cancer, earthquakes, AIDS, global warming, infection, and trauma combined, than to simply believe he is bad and I am good.

I'm not saying anything that wasn't already inherent in, "Judge not that ye be not judged."

I do believe, however, that having that scripture at hand hasn't stopped the self-righteous—meaning those who for profit or pride pretend to be righteous—from their brainless judging of anyone who doesn't think the way that they do. They won't be reading this. There are a lot of thinking people out there who don't read scripture; I'm writing this for them.

I want to address a specific issue of self-blame and guilt I have seen too often in my practice and have experienced too often myself: the thought that one should have done more. Whenever I had a patient suicide, I would be plagued with the condemnation that there was something I coulda, shoulda, woulda done differently. At the funeral of any suicide you will hear ones who loved the deceased iterate, "If only I had ..." It's the same when an accident occurs and a driver is haunted by the fact that they, except for ... would have taken a different route. In fatal outcomes the process is no different than in trivial. I couldn't have done differently unless I had been wiser, more patient, smarter, more loving, more careful than I was. If I could have saved a life by being taller than I am, there is grief, sadness, and mourning, but no guilt or shame.

The same can become true for those psychological realities. For me to continue working after a patient suicided, I had to keep repeating this message to myself over and over. For me to help one who suffered from guilt, I had to keep repeating it to them. The reality of this concept helps; it just doesn't come naturally to those (all) of us raised with the BS. We have to repeat it by rote to free ourselves from the infantile omnipotent expectations that we should be more than we are if anything in our universe is amiss.

When I would treat a patient with serious shame or guilt, I would urge them to increase their awareness—purposely dwell on—their sadness and anger and grief to replace the shame or guilt. When something awful happens we have to feel something. Sadness, anger, and grief are the appropriate feelings which will not damage our psyche if we can keep (by using the logic in this chapter) the shame and guilt at bay.

12

Fear Is About It–Anxiety Is About You

I'M CHANGING FONT because this next portion is an aside—one which is necessary to make sense of depression (chapter 13) and anxiety. All that I am writing about the effect of Bullshit on happiness does not deny in any way that anxiety and depression have a biochemical, neurological basis. It is clear one's individual propensity for these physical influences on the mind is genetically inherited as well as psychologically conditioned. I want now to expound upon this seemingly self-contradictory noncontradiction.

One can be trained back at the beginning to be prone to anxiety and/or depression to a degree that will vary with each individual. Also, one can genetically inherit a body with a touchy or a resistant biological system. I'm going to describe what happens between the two modalities (nurture and nature) in an obscenely oversimplified—but I hope helpful—way.

Feeling pride actually causes a different chemical state than does feeling shame. Fearfulness puts one in an altered physical state from feeling safe. This paragraph could go on and on, but I promised oversimplification. You do the math: how many different emotions can you attach to stomach pain, hives, blushing, rash, quickened heart beat, altered blood pressure, sweating, piloerection, penile erection, vaginal lubrication, bronchial constriction, respiratory rate, urgent micturition, delayed micturition, diarrhea, constipation, trembling, vocal chord dysfunction, state of consciousness, fainting, body odor, etc.

When a thought triggers an emotion, triggers a biological change, triggers more thoughts, triggers fear, triggers more chemical changes, triggers more fear, we have a situation—a situation which I am not going to lay only on Bullshit. But the chain of events will break if any link is weak enough.

Understanding and ridding oneself of BS alters the progression. If I think you are mad at me and that causes me to be sad, I will have the biological changes caused by sadness. If I think you are mad at me and that causes shame or guilt, I will have the biological changes associated with depression (see chapter 13).

If I think I may be fired and that causes concern about losing my house, I will have the biology of fear. If I think I may be fired and that causes concern about losing my self respect that will bring on the biology of anxiety or depression. Almost always, the thought of being financially challenged will cause both fear of the realities and anxiety about the loss of self-esteem. When I would have a patient come to me for the treatment of anxiety, in addition to what medical intervention might be appropriate, I would see it as my job to help—teach—that person to dwell more in the fear of the reality but to work very hard to not think less of themselves no matter what happens. That may sound superficially silly, but martyrs will go gladly to their deaths if they can be proud of themselves, and suicidals would rather die than live in shame. The presence or absence of shame or pride can be important to life itself at those moments. The "situation" referred to two paragraphs up may well be a panic attack or a generalized anxiety state or a biological depression. If one has a normal or a touchy biological system, one would do well to be medicated in the case of generalized anxiety or depression. Panic attacks respond to medicines and to education. A combined approach is usually best. This has more to do with how physically sensitive one's system is than with one's intelligence, though both are important.

More hairsplitting here, but this is a process in becoming a happier person. Fear, by itself, is not so much a handicap to being happy as is anxiety. If I'm afraid of you, I can actually be a happy person who is afraid of something. I cannot be happy at the same time I am afraid if I will hate myself for making the wrong decision about the threat you present me or if I'm ashamed of being afraid.

A professor told me he was fearful he had not saved enough money for retirement. He was actually anxious. He was having trouble sleeping, and he was not happy. The money was becoming an obsession as he neared the age at which he expected to retire. He saw no point in talking about the problem to me, his psychiatrist, as the problem was real, not neurotic. Something made him talk about it just the same. I told him he wasn't afraid of going broke as much as he was afraid of what he would think of himself (anxious) if he went broke. He protested vociferously. We went down an inane stream of thought. What would be the problem if he didn't have enough money? He wouldn't be able to keep his house. What would be the problem if he had to live in a less expensive abode? He'd disappoint his wife. What would happen if his wife were disappointed? Would she leave him? No, she'd never leave him, but he would fear he had failed her. Oh. He would see himself as a failure. I then asked him if he would feel the same anxiety if he did some heroic deed for which he received the praise of the nation but it caused him to lose his house, thus disappointing his wife. Would he feel he was a failure? No, he'd be proud of what he did and could see no chance of depression. He'd just be sad his wife would be disappointed. I asked him to concentrate very hard on how sad he'd be if his wife were disappointed. He wryly smiled and commented it might be good to see the nagger not get what she wanted for once! We explored more for other ideas that were present in his fear of not having enough money, and they all came out to the same end. He'd see himself in a bad light. When he thought of the same losses brought on by the imagined act of heroism, there was a decrease in the anxiety and an increase in his ability to be happy in spite of his less-than-hoped-for retirement provisions.

We worked at the idea of re-aligning the popsicle sticks. Broke did not have to line up with shame, with wrong, with failure.

I asked him how much shame should have been burdened upon a Jew who lost everything, even his wife and his life, in Europe in 1944. He agreed one could experience grief and loss without shame of failure; but if he were to retire without enough money, that would be shameful. I asked him if at any moment in his past he could have used better foresight,

101

better wisdom, better judgment than he had at the moment, as he had been sure that was the cause for the anxiety (the fear of the shame). Then we talked about the shame of only having two hands if one's tricky project fell apart and likened it to the shame of not being more than one was in any parameter. I tried to teach him to have retroactive grief, not shame, when—in the past—life had thrown a financial decision his way that he didn't have enough hands (i.e. wisdom, prescience) to have handled better than he did.

I asked him to imagine he was standing naked before a fifteen-foot wall in a room with no implements or furniture of any kind. On the wall at various heights were pieces of currency taped to the wall. He was to imagine he was given permission to take the money off the wall and keep it. Fourteen feet up the wall was a $10,000 bill. Would he be angry the bill weren't at a lower level or would he feel shame he couldn't jump or reach that high?

We did a few more exercises at separating grief from shame. Eventually we got to the point that there was a 8 percent chance of a financial debacle and a 92 percent chance he'd be OK financially. We then concentrated on grieving over the 8 percent and rejoicing over the 92 percent. Subsequent sessions revealed he felt happier and less stressed whenever he took the time to separate out his grief from his fear of shame and then dispose of the chance that he would, in reality, have to feel shame. He had grief that there wasn't more in his portfolio at this moment, fear that he might run out of money, lose his house, and disappoint his wife; but the anxiety was ameliorated as long as he concentrated on not losing his self-respect no matter what happened.

Now, of course, for those (all) of us who were raised with Bullshit, this never comes naturally, but when we can remember to force ourselves to split the right hairs in the right way, it helps.

A significant, though subtle, example of this hairsplitting resulting in decreased anxiety occurred within me on a flight many decades ago from Los Angeles to New York City. I was going to Manhattan purely for fun. At thirty-four thousand feet over Kansas I was aware I was feeling my usual in-flight anxiety. I need to explain this anxiety was extremely mild, such that it would never give me a second thought about going anywhere. I loved to fly, and I loved to travel.

In recent times when airplane trips have become arduous, I still look forward to a flight as an E coupon ride. Nevertheless, back then at thirty thousand feet I'd look out the window and mutter, "Wing, don't fail me now." On approaching a landing, when the airplane got low enough that I imagined a crash might be survivable, my mild muscle tension would lessen, more so when the wheels touched down, and it would all go away when stopped at the gate. This anxiety was so subtle it would never be noticed except by looking for it through my psycho-microscope. I would have a similar sensation when innocently waiting to cross the international border from Mexico into California. It would go away when the gate at the frontier opened to let me be home.

Now, back to thirty-four thousand feet over Kansas, circa 1979: looking out at that wing, I waltzed into a memory from the time I was a child. The family was in the kitchen; my mother was reading to my father an article about a man who was killed skydiving. Both my parents agreed (probably directed at my sister and me) it was wrong for someone to thrill seek if putting their life in danger. Then my memory (airplane, 1979) drifted to winter 1956, my age fourteen. My mother, after a phone call from a friend, mentioned that said friend and family were going out to a movie that night. My father groused that they were wrong to risk their lives driving on a potentially foggy night just to see a movie. (At that time, smudge-pot-infested Santa Ana could have killer fogs–the kind that would make one leave one's car and grope one's way home.) Bingo (airplane, 1979)! I was risking my life just to have fun in NYC. If I got there safely, this was travel (always sacred in my family's values); if I died, I was wrong.

Epiphany! If that airplane crashed, I was not wrong; I was just dead! I've never had anxiety on an airplane since. I've had experiences, which we'll skip, in which I was afraid on an airplane, but never again have I been anxious. If I want to get on an airplane enough to actually get on the airplane, I am not wrong to get on that airplane no matter what happens. Anxiety was about fearing that I didn't live my life right if I were on an airplane that crashed. Fear is about the one in eight million or so chances I might die.

In treating anxiety I would often use medicine if the patient needed relief before we could make progress in therapy. I'd also medicate a patient who was sensitive enough that everyday events exceeded the anxiety threshold of that person or if there were a specific temporary stressor. But I felt it essential to at least try to teach a patient how to have fear without anxiety. Patients who were not sensitive to their own chemistry and who were bright and motivated usually benefited for a lifetime by learning to overcome the BS teaching that fault in themselves was about to be exposed should something go wrong.

One of the common causes for anxiety is the fear of missing a deadline at work or in school. This could be dealt with in therapy by helping the patient understand that if my picture frame fell apart because I only had two hands, the same could be true for the patient if he lost his job because he weren't _____ more than he was. (Fill in the blank with any quality.) No matter what it is, being Born Again means understanding you can't be _____ more than you are at any instant no matter what is at stake. Imagine a physical situation wherein I can't save your life because I'm not seven feet tall. Then you will die, but I'm not anxious over being only six foot two. The same goes for not being brighter than I am, more organized than I am, sexier than I am, more industrious than I am. Before a deadline, I can lessen my anxiety if I recognize that if the boss hired me, me is what he gets. If he wants someone other than me, then I will be fired. I will not feel differently about me if he is in Group A (all the bosses in the world that would want me) than if he is in Group B (all the bosses in the world that would not want me). Now, I want to keep the job or get a good grade on the assignment enough to work as hard and as fast to meet that deadline as it is worth to me to do so. If that's not good enough for the boss or teacher, then I will live with the consequences of that the same as if I were doomed because of any factor beyond my control.

But what will then motivate me to grow if not anxiety, guilt, shame, blame, or the fear thereof? That question always comes next. There is an obvious answer. What will motivate me to grow in the next instant is my desire to not get fired, to save your life, to have enough money in my retirement, to return home safely from a trip. It is not my fear of shame, blame, or guilt.

Panic attacks are something very different, but I believe giving up BS and being Born Again helps even them. A panic attack is a discharge of hormones (often for unnoticed reasons, though the subject may think they know the reason) which triggers physical changes in the subject's body, which scares the crap out of the sufferer, which triggers more physical change, which terrifies more, which triggers more . . . and more . . . and more. The old trick about breathing into a paper bag works because one of the symptoms is often hyperventilation, which causes a chemical change in the bloodstream and can lead to fainting. By forcing the subject to breathe stale air, those chemical changes are less severe, saving the patient from fainting so they can suffer even more.

Being Born Again can help in several ways: 1) with no fear of shame the first, unperceived trigger may be less, 2) when one learns there is no shame in the event, one more easily can say to oneself, "Rats, I'm having a chemical rush. So what!" 3) with more existential understanding the whole thing is less terrifying. Oftentimes a well-meaning, untrained helper will try to get the subject's mind off of what is happening. The exact opposite is much better. I would tell a subject to concentrate on what is going on in the body, isolate each symptom, and then realize each symptom should cause one to be pissed, not afraid.

Insight about the trigger often comes after the patient can handle the chemical event as a non-threat. The psychiatrist should teach the patient to not be afraid of the whole sorry mess but to hate it instead. Insight into the cause is not often helpful until after the patient learns to fear the attack less.

Ralph came to see me because his panic attacks while commuting caused him an inability to drive on the freeway. In Los Angeles that's about as bad as an Inuit being terrorized by the color white. He commuted forty miles each way to work. A freeway connected his home neighborhood directly to his work site, but he'd drive further with a longer commute time by using only surface streets. I treated him before good drugs were available to help him.

We began by focusing on the fact this could be helped and would be worth it. It was understood he'd have homework, which would be more important than his sessions. With behavioral treatment, I got Ralph to drive on the freeway from one ramp to the next. This gradually increased over time until he was commuting again to work by freeway. In one of his last sessions, he told me a few days earlier he had seen at the spot where he'd had his first panic attack a sign that he'd never noticed before advertising flights to the city where Alice, his recently divorced ex-wife, was living. Of course this is anecdotal, and I can't claim to know anything, but I believe his hormone system was triggered to fart when he had an unconscious association to his ex. Because of the lack of awareness, the physical effect frightened him. Then he became anxious to approach the site where he'd had an unexplained panic, and it had metastasized from there.

I inherited a body sensitive to the chemistry of panic attacks from my mother. Her life was compromised (and activities of the whole family pretty much controlled) by her phobic avoidances. She never had the desire for any insight or curing because it worked for her to manage everyone around her. She was a control freak–but that was, reflexly, largely due to her fear of her anxiety. Being somewhat Born Again helped me, although angry about it, to not blame her.

One beautiful, sunny day back in the late seventies, I was driving my top-down Beetle on East First Street in Santa Ana. The radio was playing Mozart; I was feeling fine. There was nothing in my experience to account for any stress. I was headed home from a pleasant and productive assignment when suddenly, holy crap, I panicked. Now, by this time panic attacks didn't scare me, but they made me very curious. Consequently, they ended almost immediately most of the time. Out of said interest, I looked back from the driver's seat and saw I had passed the old Excelsior Creamery, which was a landmark of the neighborhood. I had not noted it when I drove by as I was upping the volume on the radio. My very next thought was a memory of a field trip in the first grade on which my class had been taken to a creamery–maybe, maybe not, probably that one. On the tour, the guide for the group took us into a walk-in refrigerator the size of Notre Dame and scared us by secretly locking the door for a moment. That memory came back as fresh as some remember 9/11, although I had forgotten it for three decades. You know me well enough by now to know I don't know anything for sure, but you know what I'm thinking. An unconscious perception had caused my adrenaline system to act as if I were locked in a freezer. Then I had freaked that for no conscious reason my heart had started to pound and my breathing became rapid, shallow, and forced. This caused me to feel faint. About that time I'd been able to shake it off because of my knowledge that it was a benign burp of my brain chemicals. Only then was I able to see the associations involved in its cause.

Panic attacks are called panic attacks because the body responds as if it were panicking when the mind sees no reason for such chemical impishness, and one is terrified of what is happening in the body. A motivated patient can learn to be amused by them, and they–even though they may continue–will no longer be a major inconvenience. This may seem overly optimistic, and it is a very-best-case scenario. There are also now drugs that help–help a lot.

I maintain one cannot have ordinary anxiety (panic attacks, as in the above, are a different story) without the fear of ego damage. If you're anxious about your job or school assignment, about a performance, about your money, or anxious someone will find fault with you, then you're afraid that you'll think less of yourself if there is disappointment in such a crisis. The physical symptoms of general anxiety are the body's response to that ego threat. Even if you were to have a physical, chemical, hormonal, body sensitivity such that chronic anxiety is ongoing on a physical basis, it still helps some to be angry your body does this without feeling less of yourself. I might be angry I can't reach as high as a seven foot person, but I don't have to think less of myself over the fact. I'm angry I inherited my mother's panic-prone biology, but I don't think less of myself for that either. And once I understand it, it's not as big a deal as other things I inherited and don't like.

Performance anxiety is another special case of anxiety. In it, a person with biochemical vulnerabilities to such will secrete brain hormones that cause intense and uncomfortable physical symptoms when one is "on stage." Medicine is now available to simply shut off the chemical response, and many sufferers are dramatically helped by those drugs. Before they were available there was some success with psychotherapy, which taught victims of performance anxiety to not debase their egos with shame over having such attacks. They also could be helped some by specific exercises in freeing themselves from the BS and by conditioning.

By being Born Again and giving up Bullshit, one can learn that one never need fear ego loss while one does remain afraid of those things that cause fear. I may go back to my car afraid I have a parking ticket, afraid forty dollars worth. If I'm anxious, then I am set up to blame myself for getting a parking ticket. If I come back to an expired meter with no ticket, I think I was OK to have not put more money in the meter. If I come back and find the dreaded ticket, then was I wrong to have not put more money in the meter? Huh? Does my being right or wrong ride on which street the meter maid is patrolling? Or does just my forty dollars ride on which street the meter maid is patrolling? Fear in this case would evolve from my not wanting to be out the forty dollars. Anxiety would evolve from my fearing that I was wrong to have forgotten the meter—or to not have put more money in it.

A patient told me if she were to lose an expensive ticket to a concert, she'd skip the concert rather than spend the money again, but if someone were to mug her and steal the ticket, she'd go buy another. I'd project she might be much more anxious about losing the ticket than she would be about having it stolen from her. Ticket gone = blame of self unless (Shift of Blame) one can charge another. To the extent one might be Born Again, ticket gone = decision as to whether or not one can afford another ticket, letting the cost of the ticket raise one's level of care next time, not one's fear of being wrong (shame).

A few years before I retired, I saw two different men who did not know each other. There is no way their paths ever crossed, but I linked them into a story in my head which I titled "A Tale of Two Citi(zen)s." To make it more fun, I'm going to call one Charles and the other Dick(ens). They were approximately the same age, and they didn't look all that different from each other on the outside. On the inside, their neurophysiology and psychology were as dissimilar as is a weed whacker and a symphony. In reading this true tale please be advised that anxiety is stress—why else would this story be in this chapter.

Chuck came to my office at the request of his wife. She was the identified patient whom I was treating for depression, and she thought if he were involved in the therapy it would help her—at least she'd have the assurance he understood why I had prescribed the medicines. When I asked about his job, I learned he had no stress on the job at all—insofar as he could see. He liked his job, thrived on going to work, and was happy with his career.

Dick had come to see me because of job stress. He was anxious the hours he was at work; he dreaded going to work, and he'd lie awake worrying about his job performance both past and future. In spite of my efforts and my pills, his job stress got so severe I told him to stop work for a period of time and put him on disability.

In looking back, it seems to me Charles had been Born Again, at least in the area of his career. He cared very much about doing the job right, but he somehow had accepted that if the boss (or the world) wants him, him is what they get. If he'd hiccuped at his job, he'd grieve for any inconvenience, but he wasn't anxious about that in the sense of putting the value of his ego on the line. Dick was the ultimate believer in Bullshit. He feared if there were any lapse in his job performance it would be the end of his value, and there was no chance there would be any Shift of Blame. He was still at the infant stage where there would be no alternative to feeling as I did in the driveway at twenty-three (or thirty-five) months of age. There would be no childhood stage of blaming another. Charles and Dick were very different genetically and chemically in vulnerability to anxiety.

Dick's job was to hand out food samples at Costco. Chuck was an air traffic controller.

To Mike's story above and Georgia's in chapter 13, I want to add one of my own to illustrate how very unaware we can be of what is in our minds, there to haunt us and cause us pause (anxiety or depression) while we resolutely deny what is, in fact, very much there.

My father was one of the old-school physicians who worked 25/8 and fifty three weeks out of every year. I grew up with the conviction I would never put work ahead of my family, and I wanted to be with my kids for every event in their development. I chose my specialty for the specific reason that I'd be able to control my time and how much I wanted to work. I suppose I considered myself better than my father for nothing except I was always available to my kids without regretting I had less money than if I'd worked as much as he.

One sunny Saturday morning I parked in the lot at Capistrano-by-the-Sea Hospital to go visit an inpatient whom I was attending. As I exited my top-down VW Beetle, I suddenly experienced a classic panic attack, to which I've already told you I'm biologically vulnerable by virtue of familial genes. Because they really don't scare me, and because I'm more interested than most people in unconscious processes, I was curious just as I had been in the same car some months before passing the creamery. This time my mental journey went further and had a surprising twist. The first thing I noticed when looking around was Dr. Price's Mercedes-Benz SL roadster parked near my bug. My next thought was that when I see those cars at Mission Hospital they belong to surgeons, but Price was a psychiatrist. When confronted with someone in my specialty being able to afford that car, I was slapped upside the head with the obvious—I wasn't working as hard as I could be working. My father never earned enough money that he would have bought that Benz, but he always worked as hard as he could. My next thought was I'm not as good a man as my father because I'm not working as much as I could—a direct contradiction to my life-long decision to never work the kind of hours he had.

Being a medical doctor also gave me a window into the oceans of anxiety and fear engulfing many cancer patients. Often it is as simple as they are afraid of pain, disability, and dying but anxious they won't be strong, they'll make a wrong medical decision, or they'll give up too early or too late. My sister was surgically treated for breast cancer and was thought to be free of disease but was given an option of chemotherapy "just to be sure." She told me she was opting for the chemotherapy because if she died of the disease she at least would not blame herself.

Support groups are more effective than could be explained by simple education and companionship. Fear, in such a setting, could be decreased or increased by what one might learn about the subject disease, but anxiety is decreased by what one learns involving self-acceptance in the face of the fear, the body changes, the financial catastrophes, or the seemingly demeaning medical and therapy impositions.

"Fear makes the wolf bigger than he is."

GERMAN PROVERB

13

Sadness Is About It–Depression Is About You

DEPRESSION IS A PERVERSION of sadness and anger, as anxiety is a perversion of fear. That's all. You can skip on to chapter 14.

Grief, fear, sadness, and anger are appropriate emotions when something is not the way you want or when you sense something may turn out to be the way you don't want. This is analogous to how happiness and joy are appropriate emotions when you do get what you want or sense you will get what you want. We are not taught as part of the BS to have any pathological symptoms (manifestations of problems or illnesses) when we feel happiness or joy. We are taught by the BS to have pathological symptoms when we have anger or fear or sadness or grief. I don't remember any child ever being taught to not be happy when things were good. Every child was told to not be sad or angry many times when things were not good. Can you imagine a parent saying to a child on Christmas morning or their birthday, "Come on, dear, don't be happy"? But we were all told to not be angry or sad thousands of times. This was usually an attempt at comforting by one who wasn't aware that they were adding to the buildup of BS.

When my own kids were little, I tried to remember to say something like, "You should be mad. Be more mad, but I won't let you hit (or scream or throw things or kill)." I encouraged my daughter's sadness when we were forced to give up a puppy when she was five. I asked her to come sit down and cry with me because we should when we were so sad. After a few minutes she got up to go play. I'd attempt to remember the balance would be to encourage them to be joyful even if I'd stop them from exhilarating behavior were we to be in a place where such would be unwanted.

BS falsely conditions us so that some emotions cause secondary symptoms and some do not. I believe mental health is the ability to experience all emotions without subsequent symptoms, even if the milieu won't accept expressing them.

I tried to discuss with a psychiatrist friend the essence of the difference between sadness and anger. Both are real emotions; both are called for when it isn't the way one wants it. We didn't get to an abstract solution. He didn't see why I couldn't understand how the feeling of anger was not the same as the feeling of sadness. I agreed with him; I could feel the difference, yet I still don't know if they are really all that different; both are emotions and not symptoms. The closest I can come is anger may be what you feel when something emotionally painful happens and sadness may be more just loss. Most of the time when we feel one of those emotions we will actually feel both. At any rate, I'm not sure it's a mental health issue to separate them. It is a mental health issue to not feel badly about oneself when one feels either of those emotions.

I sense the appearance of imprecision here, accepted with nonchalance, when I've been making a huge point of the need for exactitude up to this point. I'm using a microscope to separate out the cholera from the water and making shocking statements about the need to separate anger from blame, sadness from depression, and anxiety from fear. I've even made the biggest deal of saying anger is harmless, the harm comes from the fear of anger. Now, where do I get off not hanging myself out to dry over my allegation that the difference between anger and sadness isn't all that important? Here's the reason: in all the issues which I'm turning into doctrine, I'm insisting on separating the healthy anger, fear, water, or sadness from the unhealthy blame, anxiety, cholera bacillus, or depression. That I stand by. Anger and sadness are both healthy emotions that can be perverted into the unhealthy symptoms of blame, depression, or shame because of the BS fallacy. Where to draw the line between anger and sadness isn't that crucial.

They are both in the healthy category that BS falsely taught us to fear, and being Born Again is to no longer fear either sadness or anger.

As in chapter 12 with anxiety, I'm going back into the aside mode for depression. Depression can be a serious biochemical catastrophe for which it is malpractice to not attempt medical intervention. Vulnerability to depression, as such, is genetically inherited. It is about as possible to talk someone out of a serious biological depression as it is to talk someone out of a myocardial infarction. Depression can be a fatal illness just as surely as can a cardiac event.

It is unfortunate we don't have a generally agreed upon term to distinguish the above from what we feel when we blame ourselves for being sad. Sometimes those of us in the business would talk about Depression being different from depression. That's too subtle to put much trust in. However, we do use the same word to describe the force that causes a drop of red wine to fall upon a white dress as we use to describe the force that keeps planets and stars in their orbits. Perhaps we just need to understand what goes on microscopically goes on cosmically in depression as well as with gravity. Even the tendency toward lower case depression likely has something genetically in common with upper case Depression.

A depressed thought, often so fleeting as to not be noticed, can trigger the biology of depression, which can then cause thoughts so disturbed as to be psychotic, which can then cause a biological storm that a patient may not survive in the case of suicide or malnutrition or exhaustion.

Someone with the certainty of intractable pain and imminent demise who elects euthanasia is often not suicidal. They are not wanting to die; they are merely controlling the event. Real suicide is caused by depression, a delusional depression. One doesn't kill oneself over a financial desperation, but the financial desperation may cause a depression that kills. Ditto for infidelity, some drugs in the brain, the fear of prosecution, terminal illness, etc.

This last point is not understood in our society, and it's not being addressed adequately in spite of the public service announcements trying to educate about mental illness. The news often reports suicides with the suspicion of an external cause—a legal problem, marital distress, a health crisis, or financial collapse. Even what may appear to meet my definition as euthanasia may not be so. Public service announcements warn of the dire consequences of untreated depression. It seems as though the left hand doesn't know what the right hand is doing in the case of this publicity. Depression kills. Events don't cause suicide unless they are the trigger for depression. A terminal illness may motivate one patient to make the most of every moment. In another it may spawn a depression leading to suicide, although the event may be reported as self-euthanasia. To be better educators in our attempts to save people from suicide, we need to be teaching suicide is not a reaction to the problems faced by the victim; it is the result of a usually treatable depression. Perhaps the suicides related to Bernie Madoff's schemes and the death of Robin Williams are examples of fatal depression, although the messages from the press were more likely to make readers think of these as reactions to financial ruin and public embarrassment in the former cases and a disabling illness in the latter.

Gun control advocates preach guns kill people; their opponents say people kill people using guns. Either way, reporting suicides in newsworthy cases without mentioning the depression is like reporting mass murders in schools without mentioning the guns. I don't know the solution to this. It is proper for journalists to convey the news. It is not proper for them to convey speculation or to make diagnoses. For them to report that a certain person suicided is telling the news. For them to be claiming the decedent died of depression would not be proper as that would call for speculation or diagnosis; but most of the time that is exactly what did happen. I fear when the media reports on a suicide victim who was facing dire circumstances, it may convey to the populace that suicide is what one does in such circumstances. If so, this would be a public health disservice. It needs to be promulgated that dire circumstances don't cause suicide without first causing an illness, a treatable illness—Depression.

Let's turn our attention to simple depressed thoughts that arise from "anger turned inward" but do not advance to the calamities cited above. Remember, my postulation about BS is it makes me feel badly about me whenever something is not the way I want. The Shift of Blame offering an alternative to depression doesn't occur only in examples where there is another person involved. But in a situation where the disappointment or disaster is a one person event depression is more likely to happen unless one is pretty loose in their blaming. Examples: If I'm shortchanged by a cashier in a store, I may find it pretty easy to avoid depression by blaming the clerk, although I could still blame myself for not being more observant. If I break my toe on a normal, visible curb, I'm more likely to just be stuck with seeing myself as to blame. But there are those who, nevertheless, would blame the city for building the curb or another person for causing a distraction, etc. We all know people who characteristically will blame themselves, others who typically blame others, some who pretty much mix it up fifty-fifty. But everybody is somewhere on the balance of blame if one believes the BS and SOB of childhood.

Psychotherapy for this type of depression becomes straightforward when the psychiatrist understands it is their job to help the patient find the unconscious self-blame and then teach the rebirth of grieving or being angry without the self-reproach, which was only the result of Bull-shit (i.e. I'm a perfect example of me at this moment: If I'm angry, that's as it should be—anger without shame, without blame).

Let's apply the paragraph just above to the broke-my-toe-on-the-curb example. Guy is hob-bling around the next day, angry that he's in pain, but he's also feeling depressed and doesn't know why he's depressed. He goes to a psychiatrist for treatment of the depression. An example this blown out of proportion is inane, obviously, but it is a model for the process. (How could anyone not see the self-blame cause for the depression? Remember Mike et al. back in chapter 11.) He talks to the psychiatrist long enough for the doctor to pick up that he's feeling stupid to have not seen the curb, and he blames himself for that. The psychiatrist uses the logic in chapters 5 and 7 to help the patient understand that everyone will go through life tripping and farting and spilling milk until they die, and it is only the BS that makes him blame himself for not being better at any give instant than he is at that instant.

Below are two case examples which illustrate the gamut of severity in situations in which my approach at treatment was used and appeared to be helpful. Be very aware I am not claiming the psychological approach is always useful without medication—or that psychology plus medicine always works to give us the relief for which we are striving. But, herein it seemed that using the approach of separating grief and anger from blame or shame, reinforcing the first and negating the latter appeared helpful. In other words, the BS idea of seeing something ill about me when-ever something is imperfect was replaced with the Born Again idea that shit happens without any need for me to hate me. I'm then far more able to learn (GLC, Mazda therapy) the change that will suit me—and act responsibly and effectively—than were I blaming myself.

Early in my career, a surgeon requested that I consult on a case that rendered me feeling inadequate to an extent I've never experienced before or after. I knew I was not helpless and felt neither shame nor desire to shirk; I just didn't believe my education had taught me what to do. So, I took the inadequacy with me and went to the bedside of the patient.

Christopher was an athlete in his early twenties who the day before suffered an injury that left him quadriplegic. He'd had a few hours of knowing he would never use his arms, legs, penis, or anal sphincter in a normal manner again. I'm supposed to use "talking therapy" to make him feel better! I think it would have been easier to conduct a meditation session during the siege of the Alamo.

Christopher taught me how I could be useful to such a patient when I had no idea of what I could do to help in such an overwhelming case. I introduced myself and asked to sit down. He began by gushing out agonies of regret and self-blame for what he had done the day before: he should have been at work, he should not have lied to his girlfriend about where he was going, he should have known to not try what he did. At that point I did just shut up and listen, but I saw immediately the curse of Bullshit at work (if anything goes wrong, I should have been better than I was, done better than I did). This was not a time when I was about to do any kind of cognitive therapy and teach him what I'm telling you, dear reader. I just listened.

A bit later I dared to propose his catastrophe was not a deserved consequence of his playing hooky to go surfing. He responded in some manner that is now forgotten but must have been more positive than negative, and I dared to make several more such interpretations, always on the same point—what happened to him was not a deserved consequence of something for which he was blaming himself. We spent about an hour together. As I got up to leave he thanked me profusely for coming to see him and for having helped him with his despair. He asked me to return again the next day. I have no idea if I helped long term or not, and I had no idea what I was doing, but I suspect he—probably because of his own emotional constitution—became a Superman of inspiration to others.

I am left with the belief that simply negating the false message of BS was more helpful than anything else I could have done that day. Two more times that summer, I was again called to see acute quadriplegic patients in similar situations. In my forty years of medical practice, I saw three such patients, all within a few weeks of each other. The other two responded positively to similar interventions, and the surgeons came to see me, very undeservedly, as knowing what I was doing. The hospital trauma team referred many patients to me for the rest of my career. I suspect the good things they said about me in making the referrals may have had more to do with positive results coming from the therapies than any skill of mine. But these cases reinforced my belief in the benefit of understanding that blame is Bullshit. BS is present in every patient who is depressed, and BS is present in every person who suffers loss.

My second example was that of Ethel, a woman who was referred because of depression lasting for over a year that began when her husband, Fred, was killed in an airplane crash. I'm telling this story to illustrate one point: no matter how deeply it is hidden from the person who suffers and from the therapist, there is always self-abasement if there is depression.

Ethel came into my consultation room spouting that she couldn't understand the persistence of her depression; she knew she was suffering much more than appropriate grief. She was sophisticated about psychology and knew blame was somehow involved in depression. Her consternation was fed by her certainty she was not feeling any blame. Fred was killed on a business trip he had planned, which she had discouraged. There was no way she could see how any part of this depression could be laid on any self-blame. After she went on about this for a while, she changed the subject and told me, crying now, how she had failed to show the affection she now wishes she had as she bade him goodbye at LAX. Next, she related she had not phoned him on the morning of the day he died. Then she took me back to Christmas past when she had not bought him a gift he had really wanted from her—and it was his last Christmas. Bingo! BS says if something goes wrong I will invent, if I can't find, something for which to blame myself for not being good enough.

Georgia was harder to see through. She came in complaining of depression, which another psychiatrist had been unable to alleviate through competent to the point of heroic prescriptions of antidepressants. Georgia didn't understand why none of the medications had helped as she was sure that her life was perfect, and she had no overt familial history of depression. There was nothing going on to explain it. She and her psychiatrist both believed that the illness could be nothing other than a previously unseen biological depression only amenable to drug treatment.

During her first session, she told me she had the most wonderful husband in the world whom she loved completely, beautiful and above average children, a Porsche, and a station wagon; the swimming pool was being installed at their new five bedroom, three-car garage home. There was no reason for her to be depressed. In the second session, I heard how her husband was always there for her and was always showing his love. In the third session, it was how he would always guide her, support her, and help her to get out of the dilemmas into which she was often falling. In the fourth session, the bastard was running and ruining her life.

It took four hours to uncover that Georgia was angry, very angry–four hours of therapy for Georgia to see that she was angry. The BS of Georgia's childhood included that one must not be angry with someone one loved: ergo she was hating herself for hating her husband. It was actually very easy to teach Georgia to lovingly stop her husband from controlling her. They were a lucky couple as neither needed the roles they had been wrongly taught they were supposed to play in a marriage. Rare, indeed!

My idea that debasement is always present in psychological depression appears to be absurd unless one understands that debasement can be as varied as wind that may gently cause falling leaves to flutter or may destroy lives and locales in a Category 5 hurricane. Debasement does not have to be obvious guilt or blame. It can be other things that incorporate those poisons so subtly as to cause awe.

In the decade of the '70s two of my friends experienced similar traumas, each with opposite psychological outcomes. These were not patients; they did not know each other; they did not feel they had symptoms for which any intervention was warranted, and anyone hearing the stories would see both as entirely normal–as did I.

Morita told me she had been anxious and depressed since being held up at gunpoint some weeks previously. The symptoms were too minor to note as being post-traumatic stress disorder; there was nothing abnormal about her reaction. She did not blame herself in any way. She had been walking to her car at midday in the parking lot of an upscale shopping mall. When she told me her story she mentioned the gun and said, "I was helpless." Nothing worthy of psychiatric intervention about that!

But let's use our psycho-microscope. Something bad happened; it changed her perception of herself. Morita was a self-assured woman who felt very able to take care of herself absent this assault. Helplessness is on the same polarity of the popsicle sticks as is weakness, shame, vulnerable, bad, don't like it, and Oh, Shit! She had a very normal amount of self-abasement equal to the very normal amount of psychological discomfort following the event for those weeks. However, I believed she had anxiety and depression of a mild degree consistent with having been made to see herself as helpless.

A few years earlier, Michael had been working his way through graduate school by clerking in a convenience store. A robber had put a gun in his face and demanded the cash. When

Michael told me the story, his exact words were, "Man, I took one look at that gun, hit the no sale button, and fell flat on my face on the floor." Remarkable was his ability to tell me the story without helplessness being in the narrative, even though he had been scared. He apparently had no post-event psychological symptoms of any kind, not even insomnia. The robbery had not changed his perception of himself.

As I've told the story through the years I've been met with protests, usually from women, that Morita responded differently in regard to feeling helpless than would a man. That is maybe so, but it's irrelevant to the point and maybe even sexist. My point is that change in self-perception is important in understanding the angst, even when it is all within the realm of normal. I'm not finding anything untoward in Morita that made her feel helpless; I'm finding something normal in a perception of helplessness causing anxiety and/or depression.

At a cursory glance, the two stories would appear to disprove my thesis about Bullshit. Yes, the negative experience did make Morita change her description of herself to that of helpless, but it did not happen so in Michael's case. If I believe that BS is universal, doesn't this show my belief to be in error?

I insist that the BS is universal; I maintain one would simply need to know more than is known to understand how so. In the first place, none of my anecdotes are proof of anything. I offer them to the reader as examples of how I believe the psyche works. Were one to argue that most people do not lessen their self-perception when ill happens, I would promptly admit that I don't have the statistics—and neither does my detractor. We'd have to design an elegant double-blind study and collect the data. I don't have enough years left in me to do this, nor do I have enough suspicion that my opponent could be right to interest me in investing the energy. I have the experience of two score years treating hundreds of patients with anxiety or depression telling me that accepting these concepts leads to happier lives. I do know that doesn't prove anything. Maybe they just didn't want to hurt my feelings. I've considered that— but I still think it helps.

Some people do feel more powerful than others. Some feel helpless more easily. Maybe being held up at gunpoint outside a Neiman Marcus store in broad daylight is a bigger shock than being held up at gunpoint behind the register at a 7-Eleven. I'm only contending that if someone is traumatized and feels helpless, they will find it a step in healing to learn to concentrate on their anger and their fear, devoid of letting the event change a perception of their self (OK, Freudians, *ego*). Maybe Morita was losing her stuff and feared for her life. Maybe Michael didn't really care about 7-Eleven's money and didn't see his robber as that scary.

Since I retired, a beloved friend died of cancer following a period of decimation and pain. More recently a lifelong friend suicided when his life became painful and constricted and depression became lethal, although he'd been able to hide it from everyone. My friend, in the first case, and the widow in the second, expressed a wish for me to teach them how to endure the devastation without becoming depressed. I told them each to concentrate on being as sad and as angry as they could possibly be while reminding themselves over and over to reject thoughts of shame, helplessness, and guilt. Both of these persons were of superb mental health and knew the concepts in this book. They didn't need psychotherapy, which I no longer practice since retiring my medical license, but they did need an outsider reminding them to practice what they knew. When they asked me how to do that, my advice was to repeat by rote, "Grief, not guilt; anger, not blame; sadness, not shame."

A favorite joke of mine has long been the tale of a recent convert who admitted to his new priest that he still felt like a Protestant, not a Catholic. The priest advised him to repeat over and over, "I'm not a Protestant, I'm a Catholic." The following Friday evening the priest happened to be passing by the convert's home and poked in to find the man in the backyard intoning over the barbecue, "You're not a steak, you're a fish. You're not a steak, you're a fish."

How do I laugh at that and ridicule positive thinking profiteers who shout out platitudes to their paying audiences cum victims when I then give such advice to my friends?

The difference is that rote is quackery when its purpose is to drive into the mind something that the mind doesn't accept as valid. It's a useful technique if the mind accepts something new but old conditioning makes it hard to remember. Learning the vocabulary of a foreign language is a good example of useful rote. But if I still believe in guilt, bad, shame, wrong, and blame, then rote messages that I'm perfect in every way, I must believe in myself, and I can do it are hollow and will be useless the first time that I find something for which I can shame or blame myself.

First, one has to stop believing the Bullshit (Original Sin) and the SOB (blaming another to avoid blaming the self) and then realize one is utilizing rote solely to drive home a new message one does accept, not to brainwash oneself into buying something for which a firm basis of belief does not exist.

What I'm alleging is that the cliches of positive thinking are useless unless first one has been Born Again. This means giving up the belief in wrong, sin, punishment, guilt, blame, and anyone being any better than anyone else. What one is to apply to oneself one must apply to Madoff and Bundy and the KKK, and one must give up any sexism, nationalism, homophobia, racism, and virtue or evil. So, how do I fight against those I abhor without seeing them as bad? I suspect it's useful for me to iterate that I don't kill the mosquitoes harboring malaria with malice or belief that they are evil. I kill them because I want the consequences of them being killed. I can also fight against corruption, murder, and racism because I want the consequences of those influences being diminished, without seeing myself as morally superior to those whom I fight.

14

Pride Is as Execrable as Shame

LET'S REVIEW: I'm using popsicle sticks to illustrate the way we tend to align values. If ends labeled north and good and profit are lined up, the labels at the other ends are south and bad and loss. This is my model of how we draw assumptions from the way our minds arrange polarities with us often unaware. I was reared in a very puritanical home where drinking was bad and abstinence was good. Unfortunately, sex was seen the same way. It was only good if you were making a baby (and if you weren't enjoying it too much). I was astounded when I began seeing—in movies—that clergymen drank whiskey and served real wine at mass, and the movies made screwing look like fun some of the time. Some people see beer as great and sex as joyful —the polar opposites from the BS I got.

Self-esteem and self-abasement are on opposite ends of the same unhealthy popsicle stick. The more I have worth when something is as I wish, the more I risk seeing myself as nothing as I slip to the other end of the stick when that something is not as I wish. I claim that pride and shame are both always inappropriate but hasten to add that what we commonly call pride may not be unhealthy; maybe it consists of just being happy about something. I'm doing a psycho-microscopic examination of the emotion to separate that from really being proud—thinking highly of myself because of some external. It helps my growth in mental health to be happy about my—or my daughter's —achievement without thinking better of us because the ones faster than us didn't enter the race.

Builders of self-esteem try to find something good in their followers to engender pride. The subjects will always—no matter how much they crave attention and have pride in what boosts their egos—find negatives in the picture they have of themselves and use those to lessen the overall benefit. If they're goaded into holding the stick with the pride, they also will be holding the stick with the shame on the opposite end.

Remember the difference between symptoms and emotions back in chapter 13. If we have opposite emotions at the opposite ends of polarities, the sticks are healthy. If we have opposite symptoms at the ends, these sticks are unhealthy. Sad and happy are equally healthy emotions, just called for by different stimuli. Shame and pride are equally unhealthy; that stick is to be jettisoned.

I've seen patients and friends (and myself) build self-esteem based on qualities in which they excel. Often the result is a lifetime of anxiety over what they fear were they to ever fail. In many cases the patient descended into a depression the first time they believed they had blundered something, especially if it involved virtue on which they had previously placed pride.

The symbols can be daunting, and I'd hesitate to guess what they are for any individual without examining and understanding that person. There is a superficial appearance that some Olympic athletes are devastated if they fail to medal, others are just sad they didn't win, and others are just happy to have been there. I once treated a psychotic patient being watched over in a padded room to protect her from grievous self-harm who told me she was proud she'd never had a nervous breakdown!

Victor Hugo's Javert suicided when his righteousness was revealed to be less than that of the criminal he spent his life pursuing—a catastrophic loss of pride.

If I am proud of something, then some sense of self is dependent on an external. In that sense it is similar to shame. If I am proud of an excelling son, then I will be ashamed of a ne'er-do-well. The concept of either polarity is that somehow I'm involved in the excellence or lack thereof of something that really should have no imprint on what I think of myself. If I were to be proud of my dog being smart, then I'd feel shame whenever it did something stupid. How much healthier to be happy or sad about the affection or lack thereof from a lover, the size of one's bank account (or bust or balls), one's children's victories, or the acceleration of one's automobile without feeling better or worse about oneself.

A car is a good example of an external source of shame or pride which is not recognized as such by some owners. The owner of a Maybach or Bugatti may deny that it has anything to do with a sense of pride. They might argue that they simply enjoy the excellence of the machine. That is true for some, not true for most. The way to tell the difference is to take away their car, replace it with a Camry, and see if there is an emotional problem for the owner.

If I'm ashamed of my car, then I'm implying I'd be a better person if I had a better car. How much happier I'd be to just hate the car, but feel the same about myself. If I'm proud of my daughter, then I'm somehow saying her excellence is because of me, robbing her of some of the ownership of her own virtues. It seems fine to say I'm proud of my kids, but there is a purity in saying that I'm so very happy with them and for them. If I have a child who founders, how much healthier to be sad for them than to be ashamed of them. Pride and shame always carry the risk of depression and ego loss. Happiness and sadness do not.

If the pride is about something internal the downside is even more. If I am proud of my virtue, my loyalty, or my perseverance, I am to that extent seeing myself as better than others—at least in those values—leaving myself open to dishonor if I lose the certainty of such quality and making myself a prick of the highest caliber if I do not.

How fitting that the Japanese bushido (honor code) mandated that seppuku (disembowelment) be performed by a samurai for bringing shame upon himself. That was the other end of the same popsicle stick as the samurai's pride in his honor.

"I swear your pride will be the death of us all.
Beware, it goeth before the fall."

LIN-MANUEL MIRANDA

15

Self-Esteem Is Gas

WHAT I FIND TO BE FAR HEALTHIER than being proud is to simply relate to the world on the basis of what will get me the consequences I want. (See chapter 18) If you tell me I am trash, I don't find it useful for my therapist to come along and tell me I am not trash. I find it far more interesting, useful, and entertaining to just understand that a person whom I experienced has this view, and then figure out what I want to do about whatever is happening. Sometimes it can be fun to just not relate to an attack or relate in a way that shows it to be irrelevant. This can best be done by only giving that those around me are themselves–not that I have any esteem in need of protection.

A fun example of this happened when I was immediately behind a man in the Costco check-out line who had paid no attention to his order being processed but then scolded the checker because the checker had forgotten to give some requested attention to the order of the items being scanned. The man stood there and berated the checker until I decided I wanted what would be the consequences of my coming to the aid of the checker. I looked at the ranter and politely said he'd made his point, was holding up the line, and should move on. He glared at me and actually screamed, "Fuck you." Now, my point is that my self-esteem or lack of self-esteem, what I did or did not think of myself, was totally irrelevant to the issue. The issue was to get this guy to move on, maybe with a bit of humor. With that being my wish, the natural thing for me to say (maybe to purr)—to make the point of his irrelevancy—was, "You are welcome to fuck me if you think you would enjoy fucking me, BUT LEAVE THE CHECKER ALONE!" The man simply evaporated (maybe he was raptured right then and there), and—of course—I got applause from those who overheard the transaction. That is also irrelevant, except that it was fun.

Patients sometimes said it was helpful when I would use the following example to explain the issue of self-esteem. I would ask them to describe their car. They might tell me its make, body style, color, mechanical condition, fuel consumption, cost, age, comfort level, quirks, history, dents and scars, etc. I never once had someone say, "It has wheels." The closest anyone ever came was a friend who was trying to be humorous and said, "It has four wheels," but even that distinguishes it from a Morgan 3 Wheeler or a motorcycle. But the fact it has wheels is so obvious, so universal, so expected that no one ever thought to mention just that. That's the way I find to be the most happy when it comes to what I think of myself. My self-image is of the most service to me when it just is—just is to the point that it never even comes up.

When someone says to me they like what I did, I don't need to feel better about me; I need to understand that the person talking to me is pleased. I need to react to the fact they are pleased, not get all self-centered over whether or not I deserve a compliment. Likewise it works better for me to be honest with you because I want you fairly treated than it does to care that I'm an honest person. That in no way rules out me being pleased by a compliment and angered by an insult. But while I am pleased or displeased, I don't need to change what I think of me.

Maybe if I get the approval of those from whom I want approval, I will be a free man (a jury), maybe I'll be rich (a sponsor), maybe the first woman to head General Motors (the GM board of directors), or maybe a successful graduate student (a dissertation committee). Maybe if I displease the object of my attention, I'll be shot in the street (a felon), have to pay a judgment (one suing me), go through life alone (my mate), or have to pay higher insurance rates (a traffic cop). I'm not saying approval or disapproval is trivial. It may be vital. I'm just arguing for happiness or sadness, joy or grief, but not respect or loss of respect for myself. When a patient has come to me in great pain and distress after having been fired, divorced, dumped, rejected by their own children, or convicted, I can't help them by praying with them, telling them to cheer up, or complimenting them over anything. I can help by teaching them to grieve without shame, to lose their wealth but not their value, to be alone without being lonely, or to refuse to be disabled even though they'll never walk. That might take a lot of time, but the length of the therapy is shortened if the therapist has a clear concept of what they are aiming to do.

I cringe when I see self-help purveyors manipulate their audiences by bolstering self-esteem. Self-esteem is not something to build. It is something to move beyond. It all comes from the BS, and it's all destructive—just as is self-abasement.

If anything in this book helps you, then I'm glad I wrote it, and I am happy for you. Every human formed his personality at a time when his very life was dependent on being loved by another. Small children—hell, even dogs and cats—want to save or protect whom they love. I believe it is hardwired into us to care about others and want to help others. But if you find something in this book to be of help, that does not make me think I'm somehow worth more than I would have been should I have died before I wrote it. At least it is my goal to learn more how to think this way each day, otherwise I fear I'll have shame when I realize that I could have been helping old people cross streets all the hours I spent writing this.

Decades ago I was walking briskly through a corridor in Mission Community Hospital on my way to see a psychotic patient in ICU who was pulling out her IVs and spitting at the nurses on her first post-op day—another of those experiences that made me the undeserving hero to the surgeons. I was in too big a hurry to help the young couple who were standing in the corridor looking quite lost. Maybe subconscious guilt at ignoring them was the cause of a most unkind thought that ran through my mind about them looking stupid. Just at that moment an elderly janitor who barely spoke English stopped what he was doing to go over and ask if he could help them find their way. In an instant I saw what a donkey I was; I had a microscopic —though very real—feeling of being too important to stop. The janitor showed me something that I have strived, not completely successfully, to attain ever since. He became, unknowingly, my most respected and admired mentor—and object of my esteem.

16

Good Is the Worst Thing

AFTER BECOMING a licensed physician, I subjected myself to a cabal of psychiatrists to become trained as one of them. We, the residents in that endeavor, developed a camaraderie akin to soldiers in battle. Under constant observation—except when we needed help in making a life-or-death-decision—we performed the duties that would lead us to become experts in this medical specialty. Some of our mentors were dedicated, some were brilliant, some great teachers. Others were turds, lazy piles of shit who collected academic salaries but who never could have earned a sou based on their usefulness. There were a few who would teach because they couldn't do. Some were psychoanalysts who, having been fully analyzed, were egotistical dust bunnies but saw themselves as Sigmund Freuds.

While leading a seminar one Tuesday afternoon, one of the most loved and cool of our mafia, Dr. Phillips, did something to teach (humiliate) me. I was confused. I was being ridiculed by a professor whom I admired. I was used to only being praised by teachers I admired. The ones who didn't praise me, I didn't admire. I didn't feel embarrassed in front of my colleagues because we were always being dumped on by teachers who came up in the old school—old doctors hazed the new doctors until they became dead; then new doctors became the old doctors who did the hazing for the next generation. I knew my fellows were on my side; I just didn't get him. During the next few years, I did get it. Boy, did I; I got it! What Dr. Phillips did was have me stand up and look at him while he addressed me in front of the entire resident staff. He said simply, "Dr. Schroeder, you are a good boy. That is the worst thing you could possibly be." From some of the anecdotes I'll tell you shortly, you'll see what he meant about me.

What I came to understand about my professor's comeuppance was my being good was always about me. I always wanted to be sure I was good. I wasn't thinking of others or even, often, about the consequences. If a derring-do were coming from me, it would all be about me being heroic; it wouldn't have been about a damsel needing protection from a dragon.

A half-century-long friend and beloved and respected colleague (and the very best of my earlier teachers), Jay Hoyland (a pen name), has written a stunning novel, *The Palace of Versailles*, in which a good doctor (spoiler alert: the rest of this sentence will lessen the surprise—but not negate the beauty of the narrative—for those of you who want to buy and read the book) who can do no wrong actually allows a murderer to run free and an innocent man go to prison solely because the doctor can't admit to being somewhere he shouldn't have been when he witnessed a crime—better to let catastrophes befall others than admit that in some particular he had not been good.

"Physician, heal thyself," slapped me upside the head when I read Jay's book. My example was trivial, more trivial than trivial, but my need to be good had tortured me all my life and made me identify with Dr. Hoyland's protagonist. As a nine-year-old child I had broken a friend's toy, and—in spite of the blatant obviousness of my guilt—I had lied and denied doing it. I just went with the "It's my story and I'm sticking to it" line. My victim was too gracious—although younger than I—to pursue it. To me, the badness of breaking the toy could not be admitted. Far more harm came from the lie than would have ever come from breaking the toy. My judgment, just like Jay's doctor, was woefully deficient because of my need to be good. Until I read that novel, I never understood why I could never get over feeling nauseated whenever I thought of that day. I could face the fact I broke the toy; I could face the fact I lied. I could never face the fact I was not good.

This is the result of Bullshit still buried in me. Something untoward happened—I broke the toy—and forever I had to see myself as being not good. It was the salt in the wound to the toddler's experience of the radio antenna wires in the driveway.

If I were to understand the BS and become BA, I'd realize I never was good, I just was and am, and I get to do what I want to live with having done. A Born Again me would have told my friend when I broke his toy. The consequences of paying for the toy would have been nothing. Believing in good and bad made me see myself as bad when I broke the toy. Dr. Phillips pushed me along the path to being Born Again on that Tuesday afternoon.

A lot of children lie because they are insecure about feeling they are good. Making them bad for lying only worsens the problem. Helping them to stop feeling bad about themselves for what they are lying about and for the lying itself lessens future problems. If a child's behavior at school causes a painful consequence for that child, comfort the child while the child lives with that consequence. Many parents bail out the kid and then punish them for being bad while they feel good about themselves for doing each.

In *The Reader*, Kate Winslet's character allows the deaths of her charges because she was responsible for them. Better to have people die than to see oneself as not responsible (bad).

Wherein comes the happiness of a good person who believes himself to be better than his brothers? That's what it's all about. One can't see oneself as good unless one sees oneself as better than those considered to be bad—what a colossal waste of love and happiness.

I remember when I was a child my parents were extremely judgmental of other adults who differed from them in any way. A lot of the damage Dr. Phillips saw in me was done because they had to see themselves as good. I don't blame them for that, but I recognize it as fact.

When I was eleven, the family took a road trip to San Francisco for a short holiday. We took a room at the Ocean Park Motel near the zoo where rooms were six dollars and fifty cents a night and drove into town to see the sights—including the Nob Hill hotels where bad people stayed, people who cheated on their taxes, didn't know the value of the dollar, and engaged in unethical business practices for unmerited profit. Then, on the way back south we'd drive past the fun-zone motels along the Great Highway where "dirty" people stayed in four dollar rooms. My parents taught me that anyone who differed from us in any way was not as "good" as we were.

I'm happier if people around me are happy. That doesn't make me good. It makes me happy.

If I have an extra loaf of bread that is going to get stale, I'm happier to give it to a hungry person even if I don't know them. I might have to love them to be happier to have them have bread for which I hunger, but that's a different issue (chapter 18).

I loved my work. It was wonderful to feel the happiness that would come from helping someone to suffer less. But when I'm at a place where everyone around me is happy, it does do something for my happiness that is of a different nature than when I'm around pain, depression, angst, and hurt. When people around me are happy, it's somehow happier for me than were I to be around people whom I feel are less good than I. I'd rather make you happy than make myself good. I'd rather be enjoying the life that is mine, however much there is, than waste it becoming a saint.

17

It's Not Time That Heals

IN PART 1 OF THIS BOOK, I SPENT some ink attempting to make real the concept of infantile omnipotence. If I was successful, this chapter will be easy.

Infantile omnipotence is a misconception on the part of the infant based on a total lack of awareness of anything except what the infant senses. The baby perceives nothing in the universe that has any action other than those interactions with themselves. This misconception precedes the Original Sin (BS) which is the specific biological and psychological conditioning that makes the infant feel it is less when anything is untoward in its universe.

It is absolutely normal for us to grow up believing–in the presence of any discomfort (if someone doesn't like us), if an accident befalls us, if an authority punishes us, or if a small, still voice inside us censors us–something ill about ourselves that just isn't true. One comes to realize it isn't true by being Born Again.

In case I haven't been clear enough: infantile omnipotence is a myth, a misunderstanding, a false belief of an infant's mind regarding how important is that infant. But it is the only belief possible to a mind that has had absolutely no experience. Everything that enters the infant's mind is perceived as being only about them.

Jody was a good friend. She was a French language professor who had spent some months living in an apartment in Paris. Years later she illustrated for me how she was overly prone to blame herself by telling me that after being in the apartment for a few days she noticed a large crack in the sixteen-foot-high high ceiling and immediately feared she had done something to have caused the crack. What Jody called her ever present need to blame herself was a vestige of infantile omnipotence. This illustrates my contention that we never completely grow out of anything.

To whatever measure one is Born Again, nothing is personal. It doesn't rain on our parade. It just rains; we're the ones who are parading in the rain. Mean people suck. They are not mean to us; they are just mean. We happen to be there while they are being mean. When your lover leaves you, he leaves you because he is a leaver. If she stays with you it is because she is a stayer. In my practice I saw spouses standing by their mates through sickness, health, murder, fanaticism, and other nuisances. I've also seen spouses leave their mates touting they were not to blame for leaving; it was the mate's fault for having gone bald and refusing to get a hair transplant or for getting fat or wrinkled.

It is through understanding the world (not myself) that I grow into an adult whose behavior is acceptable and of value to my milieu. If I am driving recklessly, I don't need to learn I am bad. I need to learn cars go out of control, collide, burn, overturn and people get hurt, die, pay higher insurance rates, and go to jail. I will be happier if I drive safely. If I don't bathe, I need to learn that my society is such that social intercourse will be inconvenienced, sexual intercourse as well—unless my mate is kinky. I will have better odds of getting laid—or hired or invited—if I bathe! If my mind is not cluttered with self-approval or self-rejection, I can better relate to society.

Imagine the improvement of one's happiness if one never doubts oneself but always knows there is more out there to learn. One advances through life with more curiosity, clearer perception, and better adaptation to reality if one is not burdened by risking self-abasement every time something goes south (wow, I'm abusing a polarity alignment here). Furthermore, I am never cocky (sure of my cock?) if I realize another's approval of me or what I have is about them, not me.

The following idea makes life easier, simpler, and freer—freer to find happiness. There is nothing you can do but some will love you for it and some will hate you for it. There are people who loved Charles Manson and Rasputin. There are people who hated Mother Teresa and Florence Nightingale. If I fart loudly during the quietest passage of "Träumerei" at a Carnegie Hall performance, there are those who will be horrified, who will vilify, who will be amused, who will seek to console, and well-mannered people who will make no acknowledgment it ever happened.

Your friends, lovers, enemies, parents, and children are all doing what they do. If you touch them they will respond according to who/what/when/where/why they are at that moment.

I long attributed to Mae West the statement, "It doesn't matter what they are saying about you as long as they are talking about you." In researching that now, it seems as if she and a lot of people said that or something similar. But, Ms. West, what do you think of yourself if no one is talking about you? I agree your fortune in entertainment, business, politics, or advertising may depend on being talked about, but you would be happier and mentally healthier if your concept of yourself weren't so vulnerable to externals.

I was once in a teaching program in which the only trainee who was unethical, incompetent, and dishonest and should have been fired and then jailed was the favorite of the chief of the program. He could do no wrong in that program, but he was rather quickly dispatched once he entered public life.

I was raised to respect and trust cops. I did and still do. This meant if the police were to question me, I'd be worried that somehow I'd been bad or was in danger of being assumed to be bad. If I got a traffic ticket, I was not concerned with the cost of the ticket or even what it might do to my insurance premiums. I was devastated I had been bad. Then I moved to Laguna Beach. I still respect and trust cops as a class, but I have learned some of them are just stupid, some are dangerous, and some are stupid and dangerous. One day I got a ticket for parking in a prohibited zone while properly parked under a sign that read, "Park Parallel." On another occasion I got a ticket for passing a parked car in a no passing zone. (I'm lucky. A man lying in the street was killed when a police cruiser rolled over him as the driver was exiting the squad car to go help the impaired victim.)

I have learned to go about my business as best I can in accordance with what I think my consequences probably might be, but I have learned to never expect myself to be so good I cannot be arrested. Sometimes I jaywalk. When I do, I realize I must be sure I'm not impeding traffic and am not putting myself at risk of being injured, and I realize there is a chance of getting an expensive ticket if seen by one of our public servants in blue. If I get a ticket, I won't feel I was bad, as I won't think I am OK if I do not. Since learning of the lack of practical smarts of some of our enforcement and learning that jaywalking tickets can be expensive, I jaywalk much less often.

I once paused at a red curb zone in downtown Laguna Beach when a friend ran into a store to pick up a difficult to carry item that needed to be loaded directly into the car. There was no vacant parking space anywhere near. The prohibited curb was away from the street in an area only marked red because the city didn't want cars left there; I was staying in the car and kept the engine running. A motorcycle cop roared up from out of the ether and demanded of me, "Do you know what a red curb means?" I very politely—but with a sigh—replied, "Yes, it means I'm a bad person who deserves to be punished." He actually did a wheelie in racing away without any further interaction. I have learned to use reasonable care, be acutely aware of what is and is not safe, obey the traffic laws unless there is a pressing reason not to (and my definition of pressing is fluid), and live with whatever this town's constabulary wishes to do to me, just like I live in earthquake territory and don't hang heavy objects over my bed. I am sure I will never blame myself if I fall into an abyss when the earth opens up. Getting arrested or careening into a crevasse isn't as bad as going through life afraid I will hate myself should either occur.

If I want to be loved, it makes every bit of sense to act in the way that will increase the chance of being loved by those who are amenable to loving. I can do other things to increase my chance of being abandoned, hated, murdered and despised. But increasing or decreasing my chances according to what I'm willing to do is all there is. And what I am willing depends on factors in me that are sometimes not understood by me. At any moment I'm using those factors the best I know how to at that moment. I will always be able to do better in the next moment, but in the past moment I could not have had better judgment, knowledge, patience, and maturity than I did. Your reaction to me is about you. My behavior is about me.

During my residency program, the powers that be decided to double the workload of the residents. When one resident protested that it was impossible to do what was asked of us, the chairman of the department smugly said that we could work 112 hours a week like the surgery residents often did. When another resident said it wasn't fair, he got the usual retort: "What's fair?" This went on for a while until I respectfully told the chief I was willing to do my very best to make him happy with my workload and performance; I just wanted him to know one fact about me: my family was more important to me than my career. He immediately said he saw the plan was not a good idea, and it was abandoned. I could have been fired. Truth is, my family was more important to me than my career. With a moment's reflection he realized that made me more important to what he wanted as well. It could easily have gone the other way. Which way it went would have had nothing to do with me. Had he fired me, I would never have been a psychiatrist, but I didn't want to be one enough to start out having no relationship with my family, so I was willing to risk he might have been that bullheaded. The issue turned on his degree of rigidity, not my degree of rightness.

Morita told me she could learn something about herself from anyone she met. I understand her twisted idealism and don't fault her for her self-centered point of reference. It revealed, however, something she did not realize she was revealing. Remember, from the man with the gun she learned she was helpless. Michael's mind went directly to deciding what he wanted to do about the fact that he was facing an external danger. He didn't let the robber change how he saw himself.

Until I got bored with it, I used to tell patients to imagine themselves popping up like a mushroom in the middle of a lawn. They were to look out at the world beyond the grass. Over here is a lovely neighborhood with family values that will cut you to pieces if you marry or cohabit with someone the inhabitants don't want you to habit with. Over there is a society where you will have a 1 percent chance of becoming wealthy, an 84 percent chance of being poor, and a 15 percent chance of going broke, but it has free medical care and feeds and houses the homeless. Somewhere else is a society in which everyone supports each other with a great sense of equality, but no one gets vaccinated. Somewhere else a cartel is in control. Somewhere else the weather is abominable. Then there's this idyllic community, but it's so expensive that you'd have to live three persons to a room to afford it. Out there is a place where the cops are dangerous; elsewhere the alligators are dangerous. Now, little mushroom, grow wheels and roll yourself anywhere you like and interact in anyway you choose to act. Whatever happens, just don't take it personally.

I read a tidbit on Psychminds.com this week that said, "The biggest reason the mind has such a hard time being happy is because of it's [*sic*] inability to let go and move on from a painful past." In addition to the writer's lack of command of pronouns, I'd say this advice for happiness is about as useful as telling a novice tennis player to hit the ball. How one is to move on is not addressed.

We've all heard the old saw, "Time heals everything." I don't think so. I think not taking it personally heals anything that's going to heal. The tragedies and the boons of life are things I can live with—if I don't take them personally. When the awful happens it's not a sign of my failure, and I may grieve over it forever. I don't need to get over it. I need to stop believing the BS that awful only happened because somehow I wasn't enough, and I do need to see the awful as coexisting with joy. I can concentrate on one end of the popsicle stick and be unhappy or the other end of the stick and be happy. When all is grim and I am grieving and my heart needs to be taken out of my chest and petted, time won't heal that, but seeing the whole picture of life will help. Maybe it will take a long time for me to see the whole picture.

I understand that if a SWAT team is cornering a dangerous person, they will often secure the area and then just sit for a while. The reasoning is the adrenaline level of the chased will subside with the passage of some time and the cornered will make better decisions with a lower level of adrenaline.

I might wish I were able to harmonize with Annie singing "The sun will come out tomorrow." But true as are those thoughts, it is also true that to heal from trauma, getting to the point of not taking it personally is far more powerful than the passage of time. If one does not accomplish that, then time heals nothing. We all know of people who hold grudges forever or let a tragedy ruin their life. They are people who never learned to not take it personally.

In 1929 the ones who took their financial loss personally became depressed and jumped off Wall Street buildings; the ones who didn't sold apples.

You go through life giving it the best you can at any given instant. As you see how the world reacts to what you are doing, you can change what you are doing. But, remember, you are just changing the odds. It is still true the world does what the world does.

My ex-wife was a superb vocalist with looks to match. She dreamed of a career like that of Streisand. I told her, "Honey, you can sing as well as Babs, and you look a hell of a lot better. If you are willing to go through as much as she went through to get where she is, you will have a one in a thousand chance of making it, just like she did." If my numbers are close, I do hope that those other 999 singers are not kicking themselves every time they see one of her movies.

I'm aware in writing this book that the best of books written by unknown writers have a micro chance of getting published or read, but there is a macro chance of me finding joy in writing it. I won't take personally what manuscript buyers do or don't do.

When I do anything, I agree to take whatever is the resultant chance of dying, becoming famous, being raptured, getting fired, or breaking my head. The point of following any course of behavior is to enjoy my life to the fullest that I can. I need not hang on to the tragedies as being injustices or the bounties as being deserved.

18

Selfishness Is Ubiquitous

JOAN OF ARC AND MARIE ANTOINETTE were equally selfish. They both went after what they wanted. They just wanted different things.

I consider *The Turning Point* (1977) to be the most beautiful and significant movie ever. Emma (Anne Bancroft) is an aging prima ballerina who put her career first and never married or committed to love. Deedee (Shirley MacLaine) is a wife and mother who with her husband runs a dance school in Oklahoma. The two had been classmates and competitors dancing in the same company in New York decades earlier when Deedee gave it up to marry Wayne. The drama ensues when they meet again twenty-some years later. Deedee is jealous of Emma for her career, and Emma aches for the love and family she never sought. The drama is resolved when each comes to see she went for what was most important to her and gave up what was her lesser desire.

I am again using a term, selfishness, in an unusual way to make a point to be remembered. In normal usage selfishness would refer to someone who wants what is only good for themselves. Altruism would refer to wanting what is good for others. I'm being obtuse, I guess. I'm saying the selfish and the altruistic are equally "selfish" in going after what each wants.

It makes me happier to see it this way. I learned from my father to loathe those who have more than I and see them as somehow dishonorable as the explanation for why they have more. In spite of being a wonderful father whom I respect, admire, and love, he also had a lifelong bitterness, about half of which he grew out of between the ages of seventy and eighty-five. After that degree of the BA process which I have achieved, I am a happier person to see anyone different than me as just being different—not superior or inferior; we just wanted different things. She wanted what could be achieved by taking risk, and I wanted what could come with security. Or he wanted a thrill when I wanted peace. Or they wanted historical legacies, and I wanted a carefree life. Maybe she wanted a promotion so she fucked the boss, while I wanted a hamburger and ditched out to McDonald's. Or maybe a third employee wanted to get ahead so they worked long and hard and diligently. Who got the promotion depended on the whims of the boss.

Now, of course, there are others who are different from me in other parameters. I'd love to have the brains or looks or inherent talents of many people of whom I can be quite jealous. But shit happens. I don't get to be Prince Harry. If I can accept that, then I can also accept without disparaging myself that I'm not brighter, handsomer, or taller than I am. I don't have bluer eyes than I do. My purpose, however, in this chapter is to offer an antidote to the poison that comes from looking at one more successful and attributing it to something that I can disparage. I do know doctors who would never treat a patient without knowing they'd get the highest fee. I don't look at them as greedier than I or more selfish than I; I just see them as having wanted something different than I wanted. I got what it was I wanted that they did not want. It's a happier way to process life and protects one from bitterness.

I had friends living in London who had more disposable travel dollars than I did. They came to visit me in Laguna Beach three or four or five times; I don't remember now—it's been so long ago. I remember taking them to the Grand Canyon and paying for their hotel room at the El Tovar. I took them to Yosemite and Mexico and threw parties for them. I also remember driving hours to fetch them from LAX and deliver them back to the airport on each visit, except that on the last visit I was unable to return them to the airport. I told them to please call an airport transport van for that trip. They instead conned my next door neighbor Bonnie into making the drive for them. Bonnie is one of the people I dearly love. I've known her to sacrifice anything to help someone in need. They played on this, although they were not in need.

A year later I was going to visit them in London. We were planning the trip, and I told them of a day drive I wanted them to take me on in England. They responded that they were going to take me instead to some tin-pot castle twenty minutes from their house. Also, they told me the easiest way to get to their house from Heathrow by rail, including where to change train services. They even gave me the taxi phone number to call when I got off at their station. I canceled the trip.

We continued to exchange phone calls, emails, and cards over the years. Fifteen years later they called and wanted to come visit again. While they would be with me, they wanted us to go to Palm Springs for a few days. I explained it might be they would need to rent a car at the airport, go to Palm Springs, and come visit me in Laguna Beach for a few days before returning to LAX. They canceled the trip.

The point is I wanted friends more than convenience. They wanted convenience more than friends. We each went after what we wanted. I don't think of them as being more selfish than I. I learned I wasn't getting friends by investing in them. They eventually saw they weren't getting the convenience they wanted from me. I'm angry I didn't get what I wanted. I'm sure they are angry too. But I don't blame them for being takers, and I don't blame me for being taken. Actually, I still love them, wish them the best, and invite them to visit me in Laguna Beach, but I won't get friendship by investing effort, miles, or money in them. I'm too selfish to drive more or spend more to enhance their level of convenience; I'd drive to the moon and back for a friend.

Had there been no one else to whom my Brits could have turned to for convenience, and had I no one else to turn to for friendship, we would have been codependent for as long as we would have been an item. If an alcoholic woman has no one but her husband to stay by her while she drinks and he has no other person who can supply his sense of self-value, they are codependent for as long as they are together.

I'll say more about this in chapter 20, but for the chapter on selfishness, suffice it to say the players in the paragraphs above are all equal.

*"The remarkable thing is that
we really love our neighbor as ourselves:
we do unto others as we do unto ourselves.
We hate others when we hate ourselves....
It is not love of self but hatred of self
which is at the root of the troubles
that afflict our world."*

ERIC HOFFER

19

No One Deserves Anything

A BLAST OF INSIGHT into how our culture supports the Bullshit falsehood exploded in my brain in a cinema in Hollywood fifty-one years ago. Maria and Georg are for the first time expressing their love for each other in that gazebo near Salzburg while singing, "Somewhere in my youth or childhood, I must have done something good." Bolstering my contention this falsehood is accepted without pause is a remark I found when writing this paragraph. I YouTubed the song just to make sure I had the phrasing correct, and the first comment on the page below the video inset was, "I'm now 69 years old and have forever longed to experience something similar to this beautiful scene. I know that it's a fantasy, but still hope and pray that I will someday (soon) meet my Maria. I am a very good man that deserves the love of my life to appear." Bingo! That third sentence just nailed it. Seven decades of living and he still believes deserving something has anything to do with whether or not he gets it.

When I retired, friends said I deserved to live happily at leisure in my little home in Laguna

Beach surrounded by friends and family because I had worked over four decades to earn what I had. I don't agree. One may or may not get what one earns. Deserving is irrelevant. I don't deserve any of the good things in life any more than does the janitor whom you met in chapter 15 or friends who have died within months of retirement after equally long and arduous careers.

If you hold your hand in a fire, do you deserve to get burned or do you just get burned? If you stay up too late to watch the end of the movie, do you deserve to know the outcome of the plot or is it just that your curiosity was satisfied? Do you deserve to be tired the next day or are you just tired?

I continue to be amazed at how presumed adults, playwrights, musicians, and novelists cannot get over the idea of deserving. I find most atheists are also religious in that they have not shed the idea of deserving even though they profess to believe in no judge. Deserving is a notion of BS and nothing more. At some point in the infantile omnipotence era, you felt awful about yourself if something went wrong, better about yourself if things went well. You somehow came to believe that your goodness or badness was controlling fate. To be Born Again, give it up! Things go the way you want, and things go the way you don't want.

Other than, "Shit happens," my favorite bumper sticker says, "Life's a bitch, and then you die." People get so demoralized when they realize life isn't fair! It never was and never will be. Was it fair the Pacific got to be so much bigger than the Atlantic? Is there fairness in the fact that two world wars happened in my father's lifetime, and only one happened in mine, and none has happened in yours (yet)? Where's the fairness in my studying harder than some of my classmates who were dumber than I and yet I got lower grades? And let's not even begin to consider current American political life.

To me it is disgusting to hear someone who survived a crash in which everyone else was killed giving thanks to a god for having been saved. I guess it would build my ego to think I was of more purpose to that god than all who died. What is actually happening is the speaker hasn't yet been Born Again and still believes the infantile idea that if something good happens, one must have been—or will be—good.

If nothing is fair, what's the use in trying? Well, I quite frankly believe we would all be happier if we quit trying. But don't quit doing! If I want to be loved, then I'm going to do the things that give me the best chance of being loved. If I do that with street smarts, I will have a higher chance of being loved than if I do not. If you want money, do what gives you the highest chance of getting money. If you want to arrive safely, drive the way that gives you the highest chance of getting home safely. If you want to get home fast, drive the way that gives you the highest chance of getting there soon. Maybe the guy who drives the most safely will get there sooner than the guy who opts to drive fast. Maybe the guy who drives fast will get there safer than the guy who drives safely. Life's a bitch; shit happens. It still makes sense to do what gives you the highest chance of getting what you want. If you play the odds the most skillfully you can, things have a somewhat better chance of working out the way you want them to. And notice the difference between trying to be loved versus just going through life doing loving things.

Those who try because they believe in fairness will have a midlife crisis if they start to grow up. Those who just do what gives the best chance at getting what they want will be happier.

With my patients, I'd pretend I was throwing a die and ask them to guess what number came up. Over time, they cumulatively had a one in six chance of guessing the throw because they all knew not to guess zero or any number over six. You use your guesses and smarts to narrow the odds as much as you can; then it's just what is. It isn't even luck. It's just what it is. You know what a die is; you have a one in six chance. If you didn't study, didn't pay attention, didn't do your homework, then you maybe think that a die is a thing with a hundred sides. In that case you have a one in one hundred chance. If you refuse to play, you have a zero chance. If you play the odds as best you know how, you have a happier life than if you don't. If you expect it to be fair, you won't be happy.

Punishment works the same way—the same awful way as does fair. It's a disaster. Those accused of witchcraft in old Salem didn't deserve to be merely hanged while those in Europe were burned alive. Pyotr Tchaikovsky and Alan Turing didn't deserve extermination for being queer while Elton John and Tim Cook thrive. The Zodiac didn't or doesn't deserve to get away with murder. D. B. Cooper didn't deserve to get away with a quarter million dollars. I didn't deserve a ticket for passing a parked car in a no passing zone. The problem with courts accepting extenuating circumstances is everyone has extenuating circumstances. It's just an issue of whether or not my extenuating circumstances happen to be in style this year. I read today about some jurisdiction making it no longer a crime to steal food if you are starving. How unfair that Jean Valjean couldn't have lived there now.

Let's get back to reality. Your child doesn't deserve to be punished—ever. Neither does your dog. If you live with this in dealing with your children and your pets, you and they will be happier. So what do you do with your kid when they run in the street? I don't know what you do, but you figure out what is most likely to teach them to never run in the street again. Or maybe you watch them more closely so they don't. Maybe they can't play in the front yard until they are older. Maybe you beat the hell out of them. Ouch. But, whatever you do, you make sure your motive is to figure out what will protect the child. You do not punish them for being bad. Maybe it's as simple as grabbing their hand and saying you will not let them be in the yard out of your arms reach until they comprehend more because you love and want to protect them instead of saying that they are bad to run in the street. If you've told them repeatedly and they disobey you, they still are not being bad. They are using a neurological system you don't understand and progressing through the day without judgment or street smarts. They have a need to express their control and can't yet control that need. They might think it's fun to tease you. We could list possible motives for pages, but there is no need to imagine them to be bad.

OK, confession here: I know none of the above can work until the kid has grown well beyond infancy. That's the thing about BS. Unless you do it (the BS) to your kid, they won't live to be three. But I want to drive home the idea you (when you react in a way that a child interprets as meaning they were bad) are lying to the kid to keep the kid alive—as you should. My point is it is a lie; the kid is never bad, and we need to be Born Again and give up the leverage of the BS as soon as we can, not as late as we can.

If a child at "that age" smears shit all over the walls, they should not learn that they were bad—or that they did a bad thing. They should be praised for their inventiveness, creativity, and artistic expression and then educated it is your wall and you won't let them do that. This can't be done with an infant or toddler. That's why BS is universal.

I am totally against hitting a child, ever. But were you to believe in spanking the child, the interpretation of the spanking must be you are a mean, violent bastard who doesn't know how to parent—not that they are bad.

Punishment is never appropriate. Never. A professor of criminology whom I know well, Dave Jr., coined the phrase, "You cannot simultaneously punish and prevent violent crime." What you do to punish crime is the opposite of what you do to prevent crime. He thinks what I aver works for children also works for society at large.

While awaiting a table at a local Claim Jumper, I witnessed a mind-boggling drama of how BS affects a child while adults just don't get what they are doing. Cast: Party also awaiting a table—Mother, Father, Child, Couple without Child, and Toy. Plot line: Child wants Toy, which is in Mother's purse. Action: Mother elicits promise from Child that Child will not put Toy on floor. Child so promises. Mother gives Toy to Child. Child puts Toy on floor. Mother grabs Child, scolds Child, and puts Toy back in her purse. Conversation resumes between Mother, Father, and Couple without Child. Mother is continuously interrupted by Child who wants return of Toy. After scolding Child for being so bad as to interrupt her repeatedly, Mother returns Toy to Child again extracting promise that Toy will not go on floor. Toy immediately goes onto floor and then into Child's mouth. Child is now scolded, shamed, blamed, punished, and made to believe Mother is good and Child is bad.

If Child is reading this book, the following is my instruction at how to be Born Again and become a happier person. Imagine if the tale had happened this way: Mother is phobic about germs and won't give Toy to Child. Child fusses, and Mother finds some way to distract Child so she can go on with conversation with Father and Couple without Child. Or else, Mother gives Toy to Child and realizes the kid is going to get some germs off the floor (the toy was a toy car, for gosh sake). Child plays quietly with car on the floor, and Mother assumes germ load is tolerable and a small price to pay for her conversation with Father and Couple without Child.

So, if you see Child (and in this sentence, I use Child as an exemplar for any who feel guilt or shame when scolded) remind Child that they were a perfect child and Mother was a perfect mother. They had not been taught about germs, and she had not been taught about governance. Shit happens. Get on with life, but get over your belief you were ever a bad child, and get over the need to defend yourself by calling her a bitch.

The last time I was called to jury duty, the despicable show in the jury room was equal to the fiasco of the toy Ferrari on the restaurant floor. The defendant had been judged guilty with special circumstances in a gang killing, but the original trial jury couldn't decide whether to lock the guy up forever with no possibility of parole or to off him. The new trial was for the sole purpose of denying or granting the prosecution permission to kill the guy. Prior to entering the courtroom, the prospective jurors were given a questionnaire to complete. On it I checked the box that identified me as someone who would consider executing a criminal. When the jury pool had been educated about the case, it was polled to discover any potentials who could not, under any circumstances, vote for death. I was one who could not; talk about being a lightning rod in a thunderstorm! I got grilled for my inconsistency in front of the hundreds (actually) of potential jurors. I simply and respectfully stated that the questionnaire was theoretical; the polling in the jury room was practical. The conditions for which I could in theory vote for killing a criminal did not exist in California. I was asked to explain. I averred that I could vote for an execution if there were evidence it would save the lives of potential victims. No one was alleging this to be the case. The prosecution was simply arguing that this defendant deserved for us to kill him. The laws of California call for this. Under no circumstances could I vote for that. I was dismissed, and the defendant was sent to death row.

I do see it as equivalent to kill a man because he murdered or to shame a child for playing with a toy on the floor in one significant sense. Neither does anything except to take the sponsor of the grief off the hook and allow self-righteous posturing along with an absence of rational thought to persist. Our nation will not do the obvious to lower violence, and Mother couldn't just comfort Child while she did what she needed to do about the toy supercar. Now, I'm not blaming Mother or national politics. It's not blamable that we're not yet grown up, Born Again. It's only tragic.

If you got that, don't read this paragraph. It's repetitious. Our nation doesn't know what to do about the fact it allows unstable people with weak egos and no impulse control to get stuck in situations that go far beyond what the individual is capable of resolving and also allows them access to handguns. When the obvious happens, the problem is seen as the badness of the unstable person, and society then imprisons or kills them. We have a degree of income inequity which is clearly a direct component of social unrest. It's too political an issue for anyone to have an answer. I'm neither a sociologist nor an economist, and I don't know how to fix it. So, what we do is vilify and punish those other people who don't know what to do either but think they are fixing something by causing trouble. In the Great Depression, no one knew how to fix the economy. Hitler saw it as his chance to grab power by blaming and killing Jews. Roosevelt had a different approach to the problem—and there are those, still today, who blame Roosevelt for what he did as surely (even if less severely) as others blame Hitler. In the Claim Jumper, Mother didn't know how to handle her need to be social with her friends and at the same time calm a very normal, well-behaved kid who wasn't old enough to handle the situation Mother put on him by handing him Toy Ferrari as he was playing on the floor. As to the US political/economic system, Mother, the Fed, Cox's Army, the NRA, the Sharks and the Jets, Roosevelt, the churches, Child, oblivious Father, and I didn't or don't know what to do about anything. Some of us are stupid, some are smart, some are money hungry, some are tree huggers, some have impulse control, and some are hair triggered. We only fall back on punishing another to cover our ass because we can't solve the problem.

Don't look to me for any ideas as to how to fix it. I'm just trying to make the point punishment should have no part in the equation. If we want to kill offenders, we should do it only if we have data that it will be a step to solving the problem. Or maybe we do it because we cut out the appeals and can do it more cheaply than housing prisoners, or maybe we do it to sate our sadism, but we should not do it to punish the defendant. If we want to yell at the kid we should do it only to save the kid, not to punish them.

We are all doing the best we can, and no one deserves anything any more or less than anyone else. If my hand is not burned, it's not that I deserve an unburnt hand; it's just that I didn't put mine in the fire. If I live in a manner to take caution against being burned, I have less of a chance of being burned than if I am careless with matches and fireworks. Beyond that: shit happens!

I am not arguing with a legal system in which any untoward result has to be someone's "fault" and therefore needs to be compensated. What I am saying is all humans routinely come up against situations beyond their abilities, and that may be legal fault, but it's not reason to find moral fault with myself or with another. Einstein was a lousy father, but he fathered the best that he could. Mass murderers are handling their conflicts the best that they know how. The aim of law enforcement would be better directed toward protecting society from them than punishing them.

"So long as governments set the example of killing their enemies, private individuals will occasionally kill theirs."

ELBERT HUBBARD

20

Mistakes Don't Happen

BAD ANALOGY (but an important concept) ahead: Q. How is a unicorn like a mistake? A. Neither does nor has ever existed, though both have been fantasied and even believed in for millennia. Mistake (as a concept) has to be eighty-sixed, not tolerated.

Thomas Edison said, "I've never made a mistake. I've only learned from experience," and, "I have not failed. I've just found ten thousand ways that won't work."

Konrad Wachsmann, the most famous architect of whom you've never heard, said it with more grace and humility. While lecturing on the idea that all great architecture is experimental, he went further and said all human behavior is experimental.

There is nothing that anyone has ever done that they have known completely what would be the result. My friend Anthony chanced a slow, silent fart in a San Francisco art gallery during a posh opening party and found he had shit his pants. I bought a painting of a Times Square street scene from a gallery in Laguna Beach and later found myself in the picture. Another friend,

Steve, was asked his opinion of a painting an acquaintance had found in the trash and ended up making a finders-fee of hundreds of thousands of dollars when he put the finder of the picture in touch with an auction house that sold the piece for millions. I'm only a doctor; geez, I'm not even associated with art. The medical examples I could give of unexpected results would be of less interest but could fill volumes of boring texts. Then there was Jon, a college friend wearing shorts who fell asleep in zoology class and became a legend when he struck an eye-catching boner and ejaculated a Mississippi in the course of a wet dream.

Every moment of life, each person does what at that instant they think they want to do about what they guess is the situation they might have a chance of encountering. Every instant everyone uses the best insight, wisdom, control of temper, allocation of attention, intelligence, etc. they have at that time. Each time one does something, it will be a new experience. Tennis players say in a lifetime no two tennis balls come at them exactly the same. The thing you've done 482 times has never yet seen its 483rd occurrence—and it will be different. The 483rd time you do it, it's the first time you've done it 483 times.

There is the old saying with which George Bush had such a hard time: "Fool me once, shame on you; fool me twice, shame on me"—yet one more example of no insight or understanding or growth beyond that of early childhood. I can always be fooled! I can do something which turns out unsatisfactorily repeatedly (like Edison above) without the invocation of shame. I will be angry at you for fooling me, but I can't claim if I were you I'd be any better. Regardless of the number of occurrences, I will never be unbeatable.

There's the dictum that defines stupidity as doing the same thing over and expecting a different result. If you understand what's being said here you realize it's never the same. If I repeat an action that has time and again led to frustration, it's because this time I believe there is maybe something different. If I believe trying it the forty-ninth time will get me what I want, then I will do it forty-nine times.

Success story: Ellen was working in therapy to become less hot tempered. Her anger had caused relationship problems much of her life. She was several sessions into therapy when she told me that the previous Wednesday night she and her husband planned to attend a concert with friends whom she wanted to impress. She made the biggest point on Wednesday morning of pleading with her husband to come home from work early that evening. Late in the afternoon of the day in question, she arrived home and busied herself downstairs until about the time she expected her husband home. Minutes—then an hour—passed, and he didn't arrive. Another half hour and she was in such a state she picked up an expensive porcelain cat and hurled it to the marble floor; then she stomped upstairs only to find her husband in bed asleep and highly feverish. He had come home sick about noon and was passed out. At this point in her narrative, I asked her how she felt now about her anger. Ellen clearly had been Born Again on the subject of mistakes and anger. Her answer was, "I wish the cat weren't broken." She was sad about the loss of the Lladro, was OK with being on a learning curve in accepting her anger, and was satisfied that she had been the best she was at that moment. Her reaction after the event was an important step toward the eventual goal of being so at peace with her anger that the remainder of her porcelain collection would be safe.

If it can be seen that something is clearly beyond my physical prowess, no one calls it a mistake if I can't do it. If the limit of what I can bench press is 185 pounds, some will see me as weak, but no one will think it a mistake that I can't bench press 220. If somehow you had bet on me to manage at least 205, you'd lose your bet, but what I lifted was still not a mistake. You didn't make a mistake either if for whatever reason you thought you'd make money by betting.

But if I'm driving and I'm capable of remembering eight instructions when there were nine parts to the directions I was to follow to find your house, I will get lost and will be regarded differently than when I couldn't bench the 205. Getting lost would be seen by most people as making one or more mistakes. (Obviously I started using this parable before the year 1 BGPS.) I'm advocating seeing it as one would see any task requiring more than one's got of any trait.

The above was hypothetical, but it reminds me of the summer I was home from college and had a few dates with two different women. Clearly nothing serious was contemplated, and I was leaving to go back to school in a few weeks (i. e. no women were harmed in the making of this story). Towards the end of the summer, I took one of them home after a date—to the other one's house! There were fourteen things going on in a mind that can only handle a dozen—and we won't get into what they might have been. I've never told the story to anyone who didn't see it as about the funniest/most awful mistake a college man could make. In fact, it was no more of a mistake than is the fact I was never able to bench more than one rep at 220 pounds; even that was managed only once.

There is an aspect of mind function called digit span. Seven is a pretty average span. This means if I would tell you a seven-digit telephone number, you would be able to repeat it immediately. If given a series of digits one longer than a subject's digit span, the person will lose the whole pattern and be able to repeat only three or maybe four of the digits. They will not simply lose the last digit; they'll lose most of them. I happen to have a six-digit digit span. If you were to tell me a telephone number, I would not be able to immediately repeat it. I was on the road in Los Angeles with my son John when he was seven years old (decades before I had a cell phone), got a page from my answering service, and returned the call from a pay telephone. I was given a message to call a patient and only then realized I had nothing on which to write. I needed to move to a quieter location to call, and I wasn't even in a place where I could scratch any part of the number in the dirt. I gave the phone to John; the operator gave him the number, and he repeated it to me when I was later able to place the call. We had a laugh with our fantasies of what the operator must have told their co-workers.

If someone were to expect me to repeat a phone number, my not being able to do it would not be a mistake. If I tried because a life were at stake, that wouldn't be a mistake either. Were your life somehow dependent on me being able to clap to the beat of a song, you'd die. A kid who doesn't know more than he does about how to handle a car may end up killing a victim in an accident, so may an adult who doesn't realize his own inability to handle a few drinks. We guard society against such deaths inadequately but the best we can with prohibitions, legal consequences, insurance rates, ankle bracelets, and lawsuits. Sometimes society is as ignorant in knowing what to do about the problem as was the kid or the drinker in knowing what to do. Society needs to continue to make progress in figuring out what consequences to impose to save lives, but not being collectively smarter than it is is not a mistake, even if it is stupid.

If you put a rat in a maze and the rat goes left and hits a dead end, then goes back and goes straight and hits a dead end, then goes back and goes right and gets through, it did not make two mistakes before it got it right. It correctly did what needed to be done to find the right channel. In that process there was no mistake. If a kid dealing with the maze of confusion and hormones that is adolescence ends up shooting heroin or getting pregnant, that is no more a mistake than was my becoming far too obedient and too "good." It may be more dangerous—maybe or maybe not more unfortunate. It may cause grief; it needn't cause blame. But what if that rat or that kid go back down the unfortunate path repeatedly? It doesn't change a thing. We are all wired differently. Some of us have to go down a destructive path again and again before we get it, and maybe we die before we get it. We must do anything we can come up with to help, structure, guide, and teach, but if we slip over into blaming the kid (or the rat), we are just assuaging our inappropriate shame that we couldn't help or understand.

The first time my daughter, Kelly, used my car she wrecked it. She made a U-turn in front of a car approaching in the adjacent lane after having checked the mirrors, but she hadn't looked over her shoulder. It happened the day after she'd gotten her driver's license. That night she was beside herself with grief and apology when I got home from the office. I told her, "Kelly, there's something you've got to learn." She was expecting some kind of a driving imperative, but instead she heard me argue she didn't owe me any apology. She was confused. That's what I wanted; I wanted the confusion to drive home the point I was about to make. What I told her, after that got her attention, was if I loan my car to the person she is, she does not owe it to me to be other than she is. That includes her skills—driving and otherwise. She's not obliged to be a better driver than she is if I loan my car to the driver she is. Then she replied, "But now we have no car." I agreed with her; that was a problem. So might be the insurance issues. But there was no reason for her to apologize for not being more than she was at that moment. There may be grief, loss, liability, inconvenience, injury, but even if death were involved, she still doesn't need to feel shame that she is what she is. It was not a mistake. It was one of those things that Thos. Edison would say won't work. Making a U-turn after checking only the mirrors won't work. It was the time to put into effect my earlier comments about sadness or grief without guilt or shame.

The follow-up to the story is rather humorous, thankfully, not tragic. A few months later, Kelly was driving the replacement vehicle when her path was totally and suddenly violated by a drunken driver. Her improved skill made the accident much less severe than it might have been, but again my car was destroyed. Her passenger who knew about the previous wreck was unbecomingly agitated and blurted out, "Your dad is going to kill you." Kelly wanted to calm down her friend so she could get on with the checklist of things that have to be done in the case of an accident and blurted out, "It's OK, it's OK. My dad doesn't mind if I wreck his cars." That night we all had a laugh at her close, but not quite accurate, rendition of my previous thoughts.

A parable: a wannabe rich man went into a VW-Audi-Porsche dealer with just enough resources that it would be a stretch to buy an Audi TT convertible. While there, he was sorely tempted with a Porsche 911 Cabriolet, but there was no way he could afford it. Then he was shown a particular 911 convertible in such a horrid color combination that it was unsalable. He was told that he could have it for the same price as the Audi. The Audi was the perfect color—the exact combination which our wannabe was hoping to find. The Porsche was a real rich man's car at 40 percent off.

Does he buy the drab purple and metallic pea soup green Porsche or the stunning pewter colored Audi with the scarlet interior? The lesson of the parable: there is no mistake in which one he buys; there is an atrocity if he buys the Audi and kicks himself for turning down the Porsche or if he buys the Porsche and hates himself for not having the gray and come-fuck-me-red Audi.

Buyer's remorse is more unfortunate and painful than is the reality of having the one about which you later change your mind.

Another parable: a woman is in a burning room from which the only possible exit is a locked door. She has a ring on which are twenty keys, including the one which will free her from the frying. She may be about to die, but she is not about to make a mistake. If she finds the key on the fourteenth try but the flames eat her before she could turn the lock, she did not make thirteen mistakes.

Just for completeness, let's explore for a moment the relationship between the idea of right with the idea of factual correctness. When I say there is no such thing as a mistake, I'm usually challenged because it doesn't seem to apply to mathematics or physical facts. I see value in going through the justification for applying it to everything. If you come to agree with my point, we will both see it as inane except for my special purpose.

When my toddler grandson from New England looked at the Pacific Ocean, he was not wrong to have assumed it to be the same size as the Atlantic. A neophyte perusing their first beginner's book on modern art would not be wrong to have guessed that Warhol might have worked for the Campbell Soup Company. If you have not learned a mathematical reality, you are not wrong to not know what you don't know.

If you tell me that 2+3=6, I would believe that you did not make a mistake. Of course, the addition is incorrect, but that doesn't mean that you are wrong. If you have not learned to add, you are not wrong to come up with an incorrect answer. If you are trying to fool me, you are not wrong if you think that fooling me is something which you have reason to do. If you gave me that answer through inattention because you were watching your horse lose by a nose at Santa Anita, you were choosing to pay more attention to what interested you most. It wasn't a mistake to place first attention onto the horse and second attention to tightening your sphincters. Third priority gave my interruption an insult of an answer to shut me up.

I have found Parisians to be helpful and friendly simply by not treating them as if they exist for me. Before I last went to France, Jody taught me how to say, "I'm sorry, I don't speak French; could you please help me?" in perfect French. She even worked with me on getting the pronunciation down pat. I've never been treated so well by so many on any other foreign trip. I decided to try the German version recently in Berlin. People looked at me like I was rude and ignored me. I didn't get why until the last day of the trip when a flirting bartender clued me in. When a Berliner would speak to me in German, I was responding with, "I'm sorry, you don't speak German." The pronouns got mutilated, but it wasn't a mistake to have done my best. The cutie serving me *das Bier* well earned his tip.

"Life can only be understood backwards,
but it must be lived forwards."

Søren Kierkegaard

21

One Is Never Helpless

BACK IN CHAPTER 13, I TOLD YOU the stories of Morita and Michael who were robbed at gunpoint. The telling there was to show how feeling helpless can lead to depression in a situation where the same event without the helplessness can yield healthy anger without depression.

What I find relevant in these two stories is that Morita was not helpless. She did exactly the safe thing—basically a parking lot version of what Michael had done in the convenience store. If we were in a philosophy class arguing one always has options, we might see that Morita made a wise choice. I'm using this as an example of my thesis that an untoward happening makes us view ourselves as wrong, helpless, silly, mistaken, vulnerable, or something depressing. Be it mild or severe, it might bring one to therapy or not even be worth mentioning to a friend. But were the subject to learn to have anger or sadness without the change in self-perception (helpless), happier would be the result.

I'll stick my neck out and suppose if Morita had told me she knew she could have fainted, kicked him in the testicles, vomited on him, called his bluff, or screamed "Fire!" but decided to just give him her purse, she also would have had less trauma and more simple anger and remembrance of the fear without the anxious or depressed symptoms. Actually, she did decide that but was unaware.

Feeling powerful or feeling helpless will make a difference in one's mood and in one's biochemistry at the moment. As babies, at the time of infantile omnipotence, we are all powerful. Bullshit soon falsely attaches inadequacy when anything is imperfect. The part of the personality that is formed during those weeks is victim to the conditioning I see as a central cause of psychological problems. As we have seen ad nauseam, to whatever extent we are not Born Again we go through our entire lives victims of this BS that was done to us. The false idea of helplessness is just a specific application of the more general idea that if something ill happens we were not as good as we should have been. The infant's idea of omnipotence can yield an adult vestige as we have seen in Jody's flash of anxiety in the Paris apartment. The imposition of BS yields lingering adult beliefs that one is helpless should anything go wrong.

Part of happiness is realizing it is not a weakness when a willow tree bends in the wind. There is no defect in a toy balloon that, no matter how large, can be burst by the puniest pin. It is not helplessness that I can't be taller than I am. Then so be it when I can't think faster than I can think, can't predict outcomes better than I do, have a body which is vulnerable to gunshots, or have the genetic predisposition to addiction or obesity. In the beginning I was wrongly made to feel there was something less about me if parents were angry, if the ball I threw broke a window, or if I reached into my diaper and smeared shit on the brocade sofa.

Some of the trauma can be abated when the victims of childhood sexual abuse are taught these concepts about helplessness. One of the aspects of what makes up abuse is an inequality in perceived power. Abusing power damages people. Rape crisis centers rightly place restoring the sense of power in the victims toward the top of their agendas. Clearly, I made a lot more of the helpless perception causing depression in Morita's story than she did. Turn up the volume; it is exactly this point that is a major tenet of rape counseling. The victims are rightly taught that they were not helpless. They did exactly what they needed to do to survive. What was done to them was what another person did. It wasn't about them and didn't change the nature of their being, even if they ended up dead in the sense that what is called for is grief and anger—not shame and guilt.

It might seem this would be irrelevant in the case of a minor seducing an older participant, as when some high school students seduce their teachers. In this case the minor is still the victim. For the elder to claim seduction as a defense is about the same as defending one for letting a child run onto the freeway because the child manipulated their caretaker to allow it. I'm aware this concept might seem to infantilize some victims, but I feel it correctly pegs adolescents whose sense of maturity is flawed. The pseudo hyper-mature are actually among the most immature.

The feeling of helplessness is nothing other than wishful thinking unfulfilled by reality. I will be a happier person if I replace those fantasies with an existential verity. I can grieve over the fact I can't be Prince Harry, and if I concentrate on that grief it will not be the hindrance to my happiness it would be for me to feel powerless that I can't be younger, richer, and more gorgeous. The emotion of that amount of grief is far less hurtful than is a feeling of helplessness.

The morning on which I am writing this sentence, I awoke with a realization very pertinent to this concept. (I have long said I won't be at my highest level of maturity until the day I die—hopefully. Today's experience is fun for the very purpose of illustrating this fact and for another as well.) I was thinking about what I'd learned from the experience of having my iPhone stolen at the orgy. In chapter 11, I related how the pain was far worse than the cost of the phone and was not explained by any guilt over the activity of the evening. It had been engendered unconsciously as I had believed I would outsmart the thieves I expected to be there, but they had beaten me. I wasn't helpless, but I was defeated. With all my bravado about not feeling shame if I were to lose a race, I had lost this race, and it took me days to get the symbolism—even though I preach it.

Today I became even more aware (there's another learning curve here) of another behavior wed to worry about being ripped off, which I had disguised as being only good practice. Now, accepting even more that I can aways be taken, I'm less anxious and a happier person, even though I'm sure I will be fleeced occasionally.

Before being Born Again on this particular issue, I would buy nothing until I had comparison shopped to the point of being an authority on pricing. I thought I was just an above-average shopper; this morning I realized behind that was hiding a fear of being the fool. I had noticed a real growth in myself in three stages of overcoming this anxiety about being taken advantage of about forty years ago, though I didn't put it all together until now. The following is real but is also a model for what I would do in many aspects of my life.

Stage 1: I would decide to buy a pair of shoes and would go to South Coast Plaza (the biggest collection of retailers in the county). I would stick my head into every shoe store and would peruse those selling the type of shoe I wanted. After I had fooled myself into thinking I'd seen every relevant pair of shoes on the market, I'd go buy the one that best fit my budget and wants.

Stage 2: I'd go to South Coast Plaza and shop until I found a pair of shoes within my budget that I wanted and buy them. But before I'd leave the mall, I'd check out all of the other stores to reassure myself I'd made the right purchase.

Stage 3: I'd go to South Coast Plaza, find a pair of shoes I wanted enough to pay their price, buy them, and go home.

It is stage 2 that most illustrates how neurotic I was, how I was unconsciously obsessed with the fear of being vulnerable. It wasn't just the fear of making a mistake, it was also my attempt to prove to myself my supposed immunity to being taken. That stage 2 is of the same cloth as was my angst after having been beaten by the thief in Las Vegas. Stage 1 could be written off as just good comparison shopping prior to making a purchase, but it was much more than that. It was time and effort spent to quell my neurotic anxiety. The happiness I have found since living (when I can) in stage 3 is of far more worth to me than would be any money I'd save by living in stage 1 all my life. In fact, I'd guess in the long run my purchases have been better.

What this has to do with a chapter on helplessness is that my sense of self in regard to being the power I am cannot be threatened (well, not as much at least) by the action of another. If I want something enough to buy it, the nature of me doesn't change according to the fairness of the seller. It's just one application of the idea expressed earlier that if you kill me, I may be dead, but I wasn't made to be helpless. The substance of my being is always under my control no matter what another does.

This may all seem silly and pointless, but it is not. Getting resolved in any given patient this issue of helplessness is a major step to increased happiness and mental health. If you think I've abused my psycho-microscope with inane observation and obsession, you should see the contraptions and convolutions the European psychoanalysts constructed to romanticize their neuroses.

People commit murder and suicide to prove they are not helpless. In Vietnam and in the Middle East, America's decisions to go to war were tainted by its need to not feel (or be seen as) helpless, confusing what should have been the basis for decisions.

22

There Are No Bad Thoughts

NOIR SCENE: THE PROTAGONIST is exhausted, dehydrated, gasping, running for their life through the streets and alleyways of the Tenderloin. The pursuer is muscular, huge, half-naked with an open switchblade in one paw. In the panic to escape, the pursued rips their clothing on a drainpipe and, in desperation not to slow, becomes totally denuded when their garments are snagged again and again on the rough edges of fences and walls being scaled. Finally the naked victim is trapped in an inescapable, dead-end alley and slips in a pool of piss left by homeless sots after last call in the drinkeries of the inner city. Looking up at the menacer the victim cries out, "What are you going to do? What are you going to do to me?" With a snicker and a sly grin the fiend purrs, "Hey, you tell me. It's your dream!" A key-wound Westclox Big Ben's clangorous panic saves the rape or slaughter to be of use in a future nightmare.

When a friend of mine heard about Scalia's death, her first conscious thought was she was not a bad person for feeling no guilt that it made her happy.

That joke I told back in chapter 7 involved incest and pretty much laid low, brother, sister, mother, and father. And it was funny. I'll not tell it again because it can offend, but there is nothing in the imagery that makes me a bad person for conjuring the situation.

Dreaming the obscene, any thought crossing one's mind, finding humor in tragedy, wishing someone dead, thinking a racist, sexist, perverted thought, or any other discharge of the language/speech areas of the brain cannot measure one to be bad. Bad does not exist. Show me damaging or dangerous behavior in an otherwise intact personality, and I'll show you the results of BS, SOBs, and failure of being BA as the cause for the trouble.

At a psychiatric conference, I listened as a renowned researcher (sorry, doctor, I don't remember who you are) discussed a criminal investigation in which a rapist stated that looking at pornography had been the cause of his crime. The expert was firm in that he did not respect the uneducated attempt at an explanation by the perpetrator to be scientific data. In fact, as a general statement, psychiatrists believe the only ill effect that comes from too much pornography is boredom. Recently, however, I did read that pornographic movies can be harmful to young adults by giving them an unrealistic and unhealthy idea of how quickly a plumber will come to their house.

I remember the angst it caused me when in late childhood I learned about the Oedipus complex and the belief that it is universal. My mother was very obese at that time and oozed asexuality. I was horrified at the thought I was supposed to want to fuck her! And I could never believe I wanted to kill my father. (Decades later, my Capistrano parking lot panic attack did acquaint me with a competition of which I'd been unaware. Thank you, Sigmund.) I'm not endorsing Dr. Freud by this statement, and I'm making no claims about understanding all of his nuances even though I'm defined as an expert, but I do agree that anything that goes on or doesn't go on in one's mind is part of the richness of human experience. It doesn't hurt or mean a thing about pathology. A serial killer, an ogre, a dangerous deviant, a terrorist, or a Westboro Baptist is no different than any of us in thoughts or fantasy. They are entirely different from us in their conflicts, self-control, ability to care about consequences, and a host of other factors, and maybe they're psychotic. But if you have similar thoughts or enjoy your pornography as much as they do, it does not make you one of them.

I was once reprimanded for speaking the wish that some particular person would die. My retort was that I was not so grandiose as to think my wishing something could make anything actually happen. (It was only during infantile omnipotence that wishing something had such power.) I guess I gambled I wasn't talking to an agent of Henry II nor that the object of my loathing would become a Thomas Becket. However, let's do look back a millennium; Becket didn't die because Henry thought anything. He died because Henry said something. This chapter is alleging that no thoughts are bad. In my voicing the thought, I was entrusting a revelation of my hate to a friend whose judgment I trusted. It was no more than that–locker room talk. Speaking, however, is more than thinking. No thoughts are bad, but actions may be dangerous or harmful. Speaking is committing an act. I ran the unlikely risk that my confidant might murder just to please me.

Do you remember ever having been told you mustn't hate someone? Well, the teller is still living with Bullshit. I give you permission to be perfectly happy with yourself while you hate away. That is healthy and adult and is consistent with all mental health. Blaming the objects of your hate, punishing them, discriminating against them, or speaking dangerously of them is not.

How many times is an infant or child scolded for something they say? A most common BS reprimand is that the child should not have had that thought. I allege that happens hundreds of times before kindergarten. Unless that prohibition is later voided by being Born Again, a lot of unhappiness can come to one who is anxious over thoughts. Obsessive-compulsive persons can have such grief over a thought as to become suicidally depressed, but at that point the sufferer is psychotic. A most common psychological reason for a panic attack is the threatened emergence into consciousness of a taboo thought.

In treating patients with panic disorder, a most common scenario–one in which the psychiatrist can seem more omniscient than they are–occurs when a mother comes in complaining of panic attacks that occur when her young child comes into the kitchen or when she is carrying her baby on a stairway or balcony. The psychiatrist says something like, "Well, if you're normal, you're afraid you'll stab the baby or throw it to its death." With this, the mother breaks down in tearful relief and often will say to the psychiatrist that she would never have been able to admit that–even to herself. The psychiatrist explains that she appears to have a very common and not dangerous obsessive trait in which she ruminates over the most horrible thing she could imagine. Hurting her baby is not something she subconsciously desires. She is not psychotic like an infanticide she saw in the news. The panic attack occurs as her body is reacting in a fairly normal chemical manner to the thought, which is hiding just below her conscious awareness.

A late-teenage male told me he was in constant fright whenever he'd babysit his young nephew. He was aware he might be afraid an emergency could develop while the parents were away, but he didn't think it was that. He'd thought about every possible emergency, and it just didn't account for the level of his anxiety. He was guarded when I asked if he might be afraid he'd molest the boy, and he wanted to know why I'd ask that. I replied it was a totally normal thing to be afraid of—as also was being afraid of being accused of it—with the hysteria going on in the press. This was in the years that the McMartin Preschool fiction caused any normal person to fear being accused of such as much as if one had been a witch in Salem during 1693. Merely by my use of the word normal, what-the-hell-ever that means anyway, he was reassured into being able to talk about his concern. I was very sure I was right when I told him he was capable of being no more than a worrier, and he was just worried about the worst thing he could think of. This began what I believed to be a successful period of therapy in which he was able to work productively in diminishing anxiety, which had been keeping him from being a happy young man in many other ways as well.

One might ask how I am sure that he wasn't at risk for molesting the boy or that those mothers were not psychotic. How I know is not the subject of this book. It's the subject of years of post-MD training and experience. The subject of this chapter is that mortals have been made to be terrified of all kinds of things during and after earliest childhood. Those terrors need to be shed in order to be happier adults. One never need experience guilt, shame, or terror over a thought.

23

Lies Are Amoral –
A Commitment Is Not a Decision

I HOPE MY READERS REMEMBER Christine O'Donnell, because she illustrates the importance of this chapter. Actually, I hope no one remembers Christine O'Donnell except that I want to use her as the paradigm of those who have never been Born Again and would rather go to jail or burn at the stake than be Born Again. People like her are making decisions that are awful, and the effect of those brainless decisions is unhappiness. While running for Congress, she claimed she would never tell a lie. Challenged as to what she would do if she were hiding Jews in WWII and questioned by the Gestapo, she said that she would not lie; God would provide her with another option. The Federal Election Commission found she'd lie to benefit her financial position even if not to save Jews. She called it something other than lying. She couldn't even be honest about that.

Let's get real! Lying is not bad, telling the truth is not good. Trash that popsicle stick polarity immediately. In talking to children, we teach them that lying is bad while we tout the Tooth Fairy and Santa Claus.

Walking up to someone on the street and telling them they are ugly and smell bad isn't defendable on the basis of truthfulness. It may be defendable as a marketing ploy if you're trying to sell makeup and deodorant, but I doubt it. Unkindness is not defendable whether true or not.

It is a fact coffee drinkers have more lung cancer than nondrinkers. But if I'm using that to sell Postum, then I'm lying while making a true statement in implying that coffee causes the cancer. (The statistic results from all smokers being in the coffee-drinking sample, not from the coffee.) Figures don't lie, but liars can figure. In recent years it has been reported on the basis of statistical research that moderate wine drinkers are healthier than abstainers. Current sources claim that this statistic is flawed because the nondrinking group includes all the people who have health problems preventing them from drinking alcohol.

Francis told me he had confronted his wife with a fact that would hurt her—one he'd kept quiet for over twenty years. He did it in the heat of anger when he wanted to decimate her. When I asked him why he had done it he said, "Well, I was only telling the truth. Aren't I supposed to tell the truth?" That was a lie. He told her to hurt her and for no other reason.

That one was not about philandering, although such is often the subject of dishonest truthfulness. It is common for a spouse to reveal a previous dalliance for the purpose of making the mate hurt while the adulterer can feel good about themselves for being truthful.

A more benign but twisted example of dishonest honesty came from my mother when she was talking to me on the phone about thirty years ago. She and my dad were living in La Jolla near a cousin of hers. She asked me during that conversation if I were going to be home the following Saturday. I inquired into the reason for the query. She had been invited to a brunch that she did not want to attend at the home of her cousin Betsy. She didn't want to hurt Betsy's feelings, so she had told Betsy she could not attend because she had to go up to Orange County to talk to me on that particular morning. She was going to drive to the county line and phone me. She would then have gone to Orange County and talked to me (by phone from San Clemente). That way, her excuse was not a lie.

She burst into tears (I hadn't expected that—I was not trying to hurt her, and I thought she was joking) when I jested to ask why she didn't just tell one lie instead of two. I saw no problem if she wanted to make up an excuse to avoid the party (she suffered from agoraphobia and often avoided everything), but to go to that extent to lie to herself that she wasn't lying was pathetic.

In growing up after being Born Again, the only person to whom I should not lie is myself.

Lying is usually a problem because most often the purpose of the lie is to accomplish something that ultimately causes unhappiness. The problem here, though, is not that a lie was told; it is that harm in some form was intended or was done to another. Escaping responsibility as a motive for lying almost always hurts either the one seeking the facts or the liar or both.

If I were lying to cheat someone, I would see the cheating as the problem. Likewise, lying is usually done to manipulate, and it's the manipulation that I'd call out. Lying for the purpose of unfairness raises the issue about the consequences of unfairness. Lying will also undermine any confidence another would have in the person who lies. A Born Again person will look to what they are actually doing and admit such and determine the worth of the action as to whether or not it promotes happiness. Enriching oneself at the price of hurting others does not enhance joy for a BA free of BS.

A happy (and that includes being responsible and not blaming and getting comfortable with anger and not cherishing self-esteem) person doesn't Machiavelli. A happy person has no guile, doesn't use people, and has no desire to benefit at an unfair cost to another. This is my thesis. Accept only the part of it that makes sense to you. I can argue for accepting it, but I can't claim it as truth. And, of course, no one reaches the endpoint of growth (truth?) no matter how long one lives.

One of the famous advice columnists answered a question from a reader who wanted to know what to say to a panhandler on the street who asked if she had any change. She wasn't going to give them change and didn't want to lie. The adviser responded that the beggar wasn't asking if she had any change. The asker was inquiring if she had coins she would give to them. So by saying no, she wasn't lying; both sentences were just being abbreviated. She took it the person wanting the charity was requesting the writer to give her some change, not actually seeking data. In that case no would be honest.

I thought the column was insightfully good advice. But let's go further. What if a mugger takes my wallet in which there is forty dollars and asks (and really wants to know)—this has nothing to do with what I'm willing to give him—if I have more money on me. I either say no and admit to myself that I just lied to him or else I give him the $200 I stashed in my shoe. I would lie to any man who wanted to rape my daughter and was asking me to tell him where she was. I'd lie to the Nazi. I'd lie about your surprise birthday party. I'm saying that lying is neither bad nor good. Remember, I don't believe in good or bad except as an easier way to express whether or not I like something. If I'd like to do you harm, then I will take responsibility for doing you harm. If not, then not. How I string together certain words does not justify or redeem one from guilt—which, as you know, is also something I don't believe in. It's so simple, if I choose to take advantage of you, then I do so, and if I don't, then I don't. I'm responsible for what I do about that. Period. I don't escape my responsibility by telling the truth.

While we are on the subject, I find it amusing or infuriating or just plain dishonest for religious persons to label their faith-based ideas as "truth." I have a neighbor who has a bold "Truth Soul Armor" bumper sticker on her VW van, and from that I learned of an e-tailer profiting by selling merchandise with such a slogan. I understand this nonsense because I grew up in a church that claimed its doctrines to be truth. In that case the most conniving inventions of a bogus nineteenth-century prophet were prominent among what was labeled as truth. I am not attacking any faith or doctrine in this paragraph; I am attacking the labeling of one's beliefs as being truth. Evolutionists are honest enough to label their observations as yielding scientific theory.

We have not yet broached the important issue regarding lying. I'm not saying that whether or not one betrays victims to Nazis is unimportant, but today that is theoretical. So would be a discussion of whether or not I'd lie to protect undocumented immigrants. Whether or not there are situations in which I'd commit perjury in court, would lie to a cop, or would lie to the IRS are also not of prime importance because they occur in discrete situations. What I believed to be more vital to the lives of my patients had to do with the horrific erosion of intimacy caused by lying in daily occurring situations.

I define intimacy as being a quality of a relationship. It has nothing to do with sex any more than it has to do with buying shoes—sorry, Bill, it doesn't recognize any difference between sucking and fucking—and for a special value I want to espouse, it can even happen in limited ways among strangers. I am going afoul of dictionary or legal definitions, but I want to make a point about the relationship between lying and disrespecting the freedom, the personhood if you will, of another.

Intimacy is what in a relationship accounts for one respecting the autonomy of another. Each has equal importance as the other. My autonomy is as important as your autonomy—to you and to me. I would never do anything to take away from you your ability to live as you choose. I will never cede my living my life as I choose. I am doing what is good for me by sharing the part of my life I want to share with you; you are doing what is good for you by sharing the part of your life you want to share with me. Intimacy is not possible if there is manipulation. If I want sex on Monday, Wednesday, Friday, and Saturday and you want sex on Tuesday, Wednesday, Thursday, and Sunday, then we have sex on Wednesday. If we want a more active sex life, then we negotiate without manipulation of the other's freedom. Lying destroys intimacy because it takes away from the other the very idea of autonomy. How can you make a free decision on what you do with your life if the material on which you base your decisions involves lies? Let's say you want to only have sex with one who only has sex with you. If I tell a lie to get you to have sex with a man (me) who also has sex with the nanny, then I have taken away from you your right to decide for yourself. Even lying about a surprise birthday party entails these problems. I am taking away from the honoree the choice over what they wish to do with that evening. I'm OK with doing that for the fun of the surprise party. I've pulled off some awesome duplicity, but I'd still call it what it is.

Let's push it. If you were to tell me that you'd never choose as a mate a man who eats baby animals, and I tell you that I'm such a man when, in fact, I often eat veal when I'm not with you, I've also robbed you of your choice. Now, I do believe that anyone who would nix a relationship over the age of the animal eaten is so intensely out of it that I wouldn't want such as a mate (assuming this was not the issue of calves being treated more cruelly than cows).

I want a mate and lover who wants me knowing everything there is to know about me. I want to have the freedom to make my decision about a mate based on what is really that mate. I'm willing to let that potential mate know what I eat, whom I fuck, how much I'm willing to pay for a car, and that I will honor my mate's wishes without manipulating to get from the mate what the mate doesn't wish to share with the person I am.

I would see lying to a potential sex partner to get that person to play with me, when the truth would get me a refusal, as a behavior very much the same as using force to get sex. It is rape in denying the autonomy of the other.

I have no desire for the classic car dealer to know how much I'm willing to pay for the '61 Ford on his lot. I expect him to tell me the car's market value is whatever he wants to get me to pay. We don't have an intimate relationship, and that is understood by both of us. I will withhold from him the information that my first car was the exact model and color as the one he's trying to sell. He will withhold from me what he paid for the car and how much profit he wants to make.

When I saw that convertible for sale as a kid, I pretended I was only willing to pay 80 percent of the price, and the salesman averred I would be lucky to get it at the asking price. If either of us had been truly honest—he'd have been happy to unload it for even less than I offered, and I would have been willing to pay full price if I had to—we'd have been pretty much out of the running for getting a fair price. Getting a deal had to be more important than being intimate, or one paid too much.

Lucile and her cousin, my father, were the perfect pair of examples in such dealings. Lucile test drove a new 1960 Oldsmobile 88 coupe and told the salesman she wanted to buy the car. He wrote up the sales order, then she asked him if she could have a discount. He said no. She asked for a twenty-five-dollar discount; he said no; she paid the full price. My dad told a dealer he was only willing to pay \$5,500 (and not a penny more) for a \$6,500+ Chrysler 300F the same year. The dealer explained that this model was very rare and in much demand and not subject to any discount. My dad courteously thanked the salesman for the information and left without even giving his name. A few hours later the salesman pulled up in front of our house with the car and requested \$5,529. He'd traced my dad's license number when he had left the dealership. (I, a car-addicted Southern California teenage driver, paid the twenty-nine dollars.)

Dad shaved money off of the purchase price of the few cars he did buy. Lucile had a better marriage. Dad thought Lucile very ignorant for paying full price; Lucile thought my dad to be unfortunate for what he put up with in his marriage. Giving less power to the belief of what was right/wrong and more interest in getting consequences would lead one to be intimate in marriage but not so in car buying, unless the salesperson were hot and you were referring only to the common, sexual definition of intimacy.

My happiness is best served by intimacy between me and my mate and by an understood lack of intimacy between me and the car store, Christine O'Donnell wants to be intimate with the Nazis.

Commitment is not the result of a decision. A promise I make to another is not a commitment; it is the conveyance of an expectation. Commitment is something I feel. It is internal, whether conveyed by tongue or pen or not conveyed at all.

If I am more committed to losing weight than I am to satisfying my appetite, I will lose weight. Commitment is not some ceremony I shared with a diet plan. When I had to choose between my wife and my cars, I was more committed to my wife. I had never promised nor even had the thought I'd choose her over the cars. It happened without a conscious decision or the chance of resentment because of the level of my feelings—my commitment. I was never aware that I had made a choice. If I am more committed to being married than I am to my spouse, I'll lie to manipulate my spouse into staying with me should there be such an issue that the facts would trigger a divorce. If I am more committed to my spouse than to my marriage, I'd not compromise my spouse's autonomy even if honoring such would end the marriage.

Confirmed bachelors are not avoiding commitment. They are committed to remaining unwed.

"All great truths begin as blasphemies."

GEORGE BERNARD SHAW

24

Dependency Depends on What?

ONE CANNOT BE AS HAPPY as possible without recognizing total responsibility for one's behavior while accepting the ideas of chapter 11 regarding blame. You have to see you are responsible for everything you do and do not do and never blame yourself. When I would first speak of this, the difference between responsibility and blame would not be apparent. I would confront patients with their responsibility, and they would assume I was blaming them for the first few times we'd challenge this distinction.

The other idea troubling listeners would be the idea they are responsible for what they don't do. I'd say they were responsible for not stopping James Holmes from shooting up the Century 16 theater in Aurora, Colorado, and they would stare at me in disbelief. We'll put this together in a moment, but first I want to explain why this is so important in achieving happiness.

Every time I drive onto a roadway, I am responsible for choosing to accept the unknown risk of being rear-ended in an accident. It is a risk I accept because it is the better option to take the risk than to never leave home. Were I to get rear-ended I would be angry, maybe injured, and might miss the airplane I was trying to catch, but I would not feel that I was helpless. I made a choice, and it was the best choice, and I do not regret it. I'm sad and angry about being hit; I don't blame myself for taking that route or making the trip, and I don't believe that I was an unwitting victim. This is true no matter how tragic the event. I've worked with patients who have suffered the most terrible losses in manners analogous. I work at trying to decrease seen or unseen symptoms of anxiety, depression, blame, shame, guilt, and powerlessness and conversely push for even more acceptance of undisguised anger and sadness and grief.

Why no blame? Go back to chapter 11. Each time you act, you do exactly what is the best that you could do under those circumstances. So did the other guy. Why anger? Because it didn't turn out the way you wanted.

Let's go back to my asinine statement about being responsible for not stopping James Holmes—from the shooting or from the choice of hair color. I'm saying I could have chosen to move to Colorado. I take responsibility for my decision to stay in California. If I had gone to Colorado, I could have attended the movie that night and I could have . . . You get the point. Now this is, indeed, inane. But there is a very practical point in becoming a happier person if one can think this way.

To understand responsibility one has to understand nothing is sure in life. Everything we do is a risk, a chance. If I have the option of riding in either of two airplanes that I could inspect, everything else being equal, I would chose whichever airplane looked the safer to me at the time. I have flown on the oldest and the newest, the best airlines and the worst, and I know of what I'm speaking when I say some airplanes look much less safe than others. However, I don't know on what criteria to judge them. I was once on a scheduled, intercontinental flight on which the stewardess took a rope and tied the door shut before take off. Maybe that was the safest flight on which I've ever flown; I don't know. Back to my point, I'd take the flight that for whatever reason I thought was the safer. If it were, maybe my airplane would have a one in fifteen million chance of a fatal accident, while the airplane that looked unsafe would have a one in five million chance of crashing. If my plane crashes and the other does not, I was not wrong. I was not powerless. I was not a victim. I am just dead. I am not to blame, but I am responsible—it was I who chose to get on that airplane.

I chose to not get on the riskier appearing airplane. I chose to not move to Colorado and go to the cinema that night. I chose to not pay more attention to my fly when I caught my penis in the zipper of my pants in the second grade–no male ever forgets that experience. (I can't guess what the female equivalent might be.) We are all responsible for the choices we don't know that we are making as much as the ones of which we are aware. Responsible, yes; to blame, no.

It is always I who runs me. Always. Always. It is I who is supposed to be the one who runs me. Always and always.

Regarding dependency, I'm going to use the above principles in a specific application. It is absurd to burden myself with uncomplimentary ideas that I'm dependent if I'm a teenager who has to follow my parents' rules–or later that I'm dependent because they are paying my bills at an age when I had thought I'd be able to be on own.

To define dependency in some useful manner in reference to happiness I'm going to consider only emotional dependency. Depending on whether or not one does this, the concept is inane or is relevant. Physical dependence is irrelevant. We're not having a purposeful dialogue if we use dependency to describe the relationship between you and the utility company, braceros in the field, or butterflies flapping their wings in Japan. Defining, in this discussion, a teenager who complies with house rules and accepts financial aid from parents as being dependent on them is not a useful application of the term dependent. It is a most useful application of the term if one is filing one's taxes. Dependency depends on what we're talking about.

The only meaning of dependency relevant here is the issue of the dependence of our emotions, our senses of ourselves, and the qualities of our characters.

Let's follow a drama in the lives of two hypothetical fifteen-year-old girls who are in exactly the same situation. Each hypothetical girl is told by her hypothetical parents that the family is going to visit hypothetical Aunt Edna in the actual Simi Valley today, and the girl must go. Both girls have plans today to finally meet the guy over whom they had been drooling from afar for the past three months. Both girls do not like Aunt Edna and hate riding three hours in the car.

Girl #1 sits in the back seat of the car and sulks the whole day because her day has been ruined. She is miserable, and it is the fault of her parents that she is miserable. She makes sure her parents pay for what they did by making the day miserable for them as well. When she finally does meet her Ryan Gosling look-alike, she fucks him to get even with her parents.

 the

Later it is her parents fault she is pregnant. Now, her parents are to blame for ruining her life—all because they made her go along to see Auntie E.

Girl #2 is angry she will miss the longed for rendezvous, angry she has to ride in the car for half of the day, and angry she has to hug the disagreeable aunt with the whiskered chin and the bad breath, but she decides it is up to her to make her life enjoyable for herself. She tells her parents about her anger and then decides to cope with what they impose in what is for her the best way possible. She flirts with a few cute guys whom she espies sitting in cars on the clogged freeway, talks her folks into stopping at Universal Studios so she can go into CityWalk and find some footwear at the Los Angeles Sock Market or Flip Flop Shops, and zones into her earphones to commune with Adele.

Which of these girls is dependent and which is independent? The answer has nothing to do with her parents making her do something.

There was a horrible TV movie years ago called *The Secret*. It was about a woman who was miserable for the first part of her life because everyone let her down, disappointed her, and took advantage of her. Then she learned the Secret, and the rest of her life was happy. The Secret was she was responsible for making her own happiness. Prior to that she had tried to please others believing they should make her happy. That part of the movie I loved. What I despised was that her whole life changed in an instant when someone told her the Secret. The revelation will, indeed, change your life for the better; it was that movie's version of being Born Again. But in addition to implying that learning that Secret can happen in a moment—it took me over a year and a half to teach that to Mary—it also presented bad acting, bad writing, and bad casting. There's no danger of you stumbling upon it. You're much better off with *The Turning Point* or reading Jay Hoyland's novel.

As I am writing this, the neighborhood garage band is practicing their noise at volume all-the-way-up directly across the narrow street opposite my desk. I'm enjoying the fact that I'm privy at my age to a punk band. My neighbor a hundred feet further away is having her day ruined by these shabby, skinny, shirtless, hirsute miscreants whom I find kind of sexy. I feel as if I'm one of the girls in the back seat on the way to Aunt Edna's, and my neighbor is the other.

To be independent is to take responsibility into your psyche for the path on which you walk. To be dependent is to have your life ruined because you irresponsibly give blame or credit to that which is outside of you for your inside experiences, being unaware of your own control over those experiences. You will meet Ruth in chapter 40. When you do, watch as she flips from being dependent to independent without my mentioning it.

I have a friend whom I admire greatly. He was born with multiple birth anomalies and has current health problems which are severe as a result. He is one of the most positive persons whom I have the joy of knowing. He greets every day with, "Well, I can still count to twenty-one on my body." This guy could be in an iron lung and not feel dependent on it. He inspired me to use his twenty-one expression earlier in this book. He inspires me a lot.

When I was the base psychiatrist at USMC Camp Pendleton, I treated a young woman, Linda, who was a military dependent and also worked on the base. She was a mentally healthy woman who'd coped successfully with more than have most. Linda lived thirty miles away and spent too many hours commuting every workday. On a Friday afternoon when she was a new patient and was my last appointment of the day, I asked her at the end of the session about her plans for the weekend. The intricate detail in which she replied was indicative of her anxiety. She told me she was going to pick up her paycheck, go home, deposit the check in her neighborhood bank, come back to the base to do her weekly shopping at the PX, then go back home to put away what she'd bought. I stopped her at this point for a reason that had nothing to do with her narrative microscopy. She was going to drive a sixty-mile round trip solely to get the paycheck to the bank before she wrote a check at the PX?

When I asked why she didn't just get her paycheck, buy her provisions, drive thirty miles home, and deposit the check over the weekend, she replied she was afraid she might forget to make the deposit (wow, her forget to make the deposit—with her attention to detail, unlikely), and her check might bounce. At that point we extended the length of her session and did a little grade school arithmetic. Linda had been doing this for six and a half years, 169 paydays times 60 miles. She had driven 10,140 miles lest there should be the chance of her bouncing a check. We agreed there was a less than 10 percent chance of her bouncing her check should she skip that sixty-mile extra loop—she'd never bounced a check. So, multiplying out the odds with the miles, we came up with the fact she'd drive 101,400 miles to save the bank fee for a bounced check. In 1973 bounced check charges were probably four dollars or less.

She then burst into tears and told me her husband had berated her that she was financially irresponsible and would get them into trouble with credit cards and bounced checks. I asked if she were doing this to avoid the chance of paying a four-dollar fee or to please her husband with her fiscal responsibility. Linda was the widow of one of the very early casualties of the war. She had driven those 10,140 miles to be responsible years after the only person who had ever questioned her responsibility had died. That is not being responsible! (Of course, I realize her psychological problems were more than that—I was her psychiatrist, damn it—but whatever pathology went into that symptom is beside the point. That would be just understanding the cause of her irresponsibility; it wouldn't change the fact that she was irresponsibly going that far to be responsible.) It is also not blamable.

Young adults often feel shame at being financially dependent on parents even though it's rare to get anywhere today without some help. Let those parents put conditions on their help and the receivers feel even more shame at being governed by those upon whom they see themselves as dependent. A lot of irresponsible misbehavior on the part of late adolescents and adults in their twenties arises from those subjects having a BS- and SOB-based need to demonstrate independence. The fact they are being irresponsible to demonstrate they are responsible (independent) is ironic but not moronic; it's the best level of common sense, wisdom, maturity, and insight they have. Having revealed myself to also not yet be all grown up, you can imagine I have empathy with them, and I have no inclination to punish. I also see that withdrawing financial support or increasing the rules is an example of what we discussed in chapter 19. The top doesn't know what to do about a situation, so the bottom is blamed and punished.

A much happier life ensues if one understands what I'm saying about BS and the SOB. It is a misconstruction grafted onto us by way of conditioning in infancy for us to believe that to be responsible we must keep promises, yield to the opinions of others, obey, and always tell the truth (whatever that is). Responsibility does not demand that we follow, or that we defy, instructions. Acknowledging and heeding responsibility is the essence of independence.

The rules, bank service charges, the price of gasoline, the cost of rent, the intransigence of persons, speed limits, the robber in front of me with a gun, taxes, the price of pharmaceuticals, the rules for grazing cattle on government land, the architecture of public restrooms, Wall Street ethics, the wealth of the Waltons, Hillary having used private emails, and the fifteen-month-long construction obstructions on the I-5 have nothing to do with my independence. Responsibility demands I do that with which I wish to live with the consequences of doing. I need never act to satisfy another unless I want to live with what will be the consequences of satisfying the other.

I learned about a patient in his late fifties who was complaining to his psychiatrist (a colleague of mine) about how his life was compromised by obnoxious demands from his mother. He claimed his obeisance to her was out of love and respect, but the degree of his symptoms revealed there were conflicts about this to which he'd not yet paid attention. One day he got to the real reason for his deference. His mother was eighty-six, in poor health, and lived in New York City. He was the only child. His mother was a widow—and worth $167 million. My friend told his patient that he'd advise him to grow up and become independent. He thought he'd be a fool to defy the mother, but he was more so the fool to not see he was acting totally responsibly and independently to kneel before her for a few more months or years for the probability of the $167 million. That was an independent, responsible choice—as any choice would be. Nothing could rob him of his control over himself. He moved east, took care of her until she died, and then returned to California and bought a good portion of Laguna Beach. Resolving the myths held over from childhood about independence led to a happy result for everyone.

I guess, however, if he'd chosen to be rid of her influence sooner, he could have done so at the cost of risking all or many of the millions. That would have been equally responsible had he thought that doing so would make him a happier person. The symptoms that brought him to therapy were enhanced by his false sense of shame that he, in middle age, was still dependent on his mother.

Independence has nothing to do with who is making the rules or paying the bills. It is all about who controls my mood and who decides what I do about all the stuff of life.

I used first-person pronouns in the above paragraph. I'll let you in on some personal history. My parents paid for my education. It was a good investment for them and made for a good quality of life for me. But the scars on my soul for developing the opinions in the above paragraph only late in life have been revealed in a marvelous dream which has recurred ever since I became well established in medical practice. The dream is always set in different places with different events, but the plot is as follows: I am overwhelmed with shame and angst and agony, the cause of which is that I'm totally dependent on my parents and living with them. Out of the mire of self-disgust comes the idea that I could move out, if I only had some source of income.

Then, in the dream, I realize I do have a medical practice with enough income that I could move out, then I do have a house to which I could move, then I do actually live in the house with my family, and the dream ends with me being exactly where I actually am in life.

An interesting (to me) corollary is that as I've traveled in major cities, I will readily walk or take public transportation, but only with great hesitancy will I hail a cab. It's clear to me this is not about the cost of the taxi, though friends with whom I've traveled just think me to be cheap. I know well the undergrounds in Chicago, New York, Sydney, London, Hong Kong, Paris, San Francisco, Tokyo, Montreal, Berlin, Warsaw, Rio, and Buenos Aires. There is a real advantage that in knowing the metro system you do know the city. But that's not why I do it either. When traveling, I will never go on a tour, even though the tour often costs far less than the money I will spend getting lost, renting cars, and getting bad deals on lodging. I also thrive on traveling alone in places where I don't speak the language. I have finally come to see the reason for all of this is I'm undoing the shame of having been supported by my parents who had had to do it all for themselves during the Great Depression. Everything I've said in this paragraph is about me becoming confident that I can make it on my own. It also explains why I'm a do-it-yourselfer at home to the extent of doing electrical, plumbing, carpentry, and painting without help—even if it ends up costing me more than hiring it done.

Linda and I have a lot in common.

As you have guessed by now, during my early years I heard endlessly about the deprivations my parents experienced during the 1930s. It was all true, but the telling of the tales was also for the purpose of getting me to not ask for anything they did not want to give me. They could not say no, but they could get me to feel shame for asking. Funny thing is they chose to give me more than I ever would have asked for.

You may have thought Linda to have been bizarre in her driving-to-the-bank behavior. I've come to see that she and I aren't the only ones this weird. I've treated patients who would be considered normal by any standard who can match or exceed our neuroses and fly the airplane in which you're riding, make laws about the safety of your food, catch your criminals, and, yes, provide your medical care. So, I'm tending to guess you, too, might become a happier person by having a rebirth in ideas about dependence and responsibility.

25

Keeping a Promise Is Irresponsible

KEEPING A PROMISE is irresponsible; doing what you promised you would do is responsible unless you are doing it to keep the promise. We are splitting hairs here, but this particular hair has a lot to do with happiness.

We can agree the person who made a promise yesterday is not the same person as they are now. Today, they know more facts, have more wisdom, have aged twenty-plus hours, did or didn't sleep well, do or don't have a new virus, etc. To allow the person they were yesterday to run them today is irresponsible.

Imagine yesterday I was told by a third party you were penniless and trying to help your aged mother to pay her electric bill so that the power company would not shut off her iron lung. I rush up to you and promise to give you $1,000 on Wednesday without telling you what I had been told. I can conjure scenarios wherein such might be generous more than it is gullible. On Wednesday morning, I learn the whole story was an anecdote from a game of telephone, your mother is actually dead, and you are, in fact, wealthy. I do realize how inane is my example and, of course, you see the point. But turn up the subtlety by 1,000 percent and we'd have actual examples that have been brought to me by suffering patients for decades.

I was required to take a course in ethics in medical school taught by a learned man with two doctorate degrees in the fields of religion and medicine. Just listening to one lecture was enough to convince me that he was pompous and severely deficient in the ability to think. He looked good in person and on paper, so the fool could charm audiences into thinking of him as a guru. I think he was a stiff buffoon; 'twould have been better had he just been a stiff.

In that class he proposed a moral dilemma with which the students were to wrestle. He had made up a story about Bill and Bob who were marooned for twenty years on an island after a ship-wreck. Bob had spent the decades growing orchids and developing magnificent hybrids, which now covered the landscape. When he became ill and they knew he was dying, Bill comforted Bob by assuring him for as long as he (Bill) lived he'd take care of the orchids—both had long given up any hope of leaving the island. The day after Bob died, a passing ship discovered Bill alone on the island. Now, the question for our class of students who were educated enough to be in their second year of medical school was, "What is Bill to do?" I used dead mama with no use for an iron lung to illustrate an obvious point. My professor was actually proposing that we debate Bill's dilemma.

Orchids aside, if that's got anything to do with ethics, then I'm a petunia!

I raise this issue just to dispense with it. It is not what this chapter is about. Of course, I'm not parting with the grand and Bill is not staying with the orchidy thingies.

In our society, an honest promise to love, honor, and obey till death do us part actually means the vower honestly plans to love, honor, and obey the vowee till death do them part and will actually do so as long they still feel that way. You may hate the fact society has come to this, but it has. That is the way it is and has been for centuries. Somehow idiocy has potency such that the SOB allows Focus on the Family and other organizations of prigs of the same ilk to blame marriage instability on newly acquired quasi-acceptance of queers.

Though misperceived as fickleness, flexibility involves all mundane promises as well. If I see that what I promised should not be done, then it is unethical for me to keep the promise. It is only responsible to keep the promises I want to keep at the moment I keep them, not at the moment I made them.

I made up a parable many years ago when technology was so different from today that the story actually worked. It goes like this: I overhear you making a comment that your car is in the shop and you need to find a ride to the city tomorrow to sign papers on the house you are buying by three p.m. or you will lose the house. I step up and tell you I am going to town tomorrow, and if you're on the corner of Lover's Lane and Easy Street at noon, I'll pick you up, and we'll be there hours before your deadline.

The next day we are surprised by a change in the weather; it's cold and raining. I'm sitting by the fire with my cat, Caligula, on my lap, reading my latest copy of *Playboy* while still in my silk pajamas. I am not going to keep my promise of giving you the ride to town. I was only planning the trip because of some shopping that can be delayed indefinitely. If I have to get dressed, raise the top on my Alfa Romeo, and drive you to the city, I will be unhappy. But I do get up, get dressed, raise the roof of the convertible, and take you to town happily. I do it happily because I don't have to keep the promise I made yesterday. I'm not keeping any promise. What I am doing is fetching you from the corner of Lover's Lane and Easy Street because right now I don't want you standing out in the rain, don't want to see you lose your house, and don't want to lose you as a friend. Of course, your expectation of my arrival is based on my promise; but I'm not keeping the promise. My motive is that I care about you, and I care about the consequences of my actions. This is not something I have to do to see myself as being good.

I am a happier person if I always realize I am doing at this exact moment what I want to be doing at this moment. I will be less happy if I pretend I am being a good person by sacrificing myself in order to keep a promise.

It is a corollary that if you are doing something and you're not sure you want to be doing it, you will be happier to say to yourself, "This is what I want to be doing or I wouldn't be doing it." You might discover the reason you want to be doing it is not valid. After a certain point, realizing I'm taking the subway for the purpose of proving to the world—er, myself—I can make it on my own becomes unnecessary. When I accept I'm only doing anything because I want to, then I'm free to do something else if that anything is no longer desired. These days I take a cab unless I want to save the money—or occasionally time. Anytime you ever think you are doing something you don't want to do, figure out why it is that you do want to do it. You'll have a happier day.

Obedience Is the Last Thing
I Want from My Children

THIS CHAPTER TITLE IS AN EXACT quotation of what I said to my father-in-law when he told me I needed to start beating my five-year-old son to make him mind me. Even for forty-five years ago he was outrageous and out of date with his goodness.

It is my responsibility to keep my kids safe, get them educated, vaccinate them, and do what I must to maintain control over certain things until they come to the gate of responsibility based on their experience and knowledge. But what I want for them is that they care what happens to them and develop the good sense and wisdom to understand the likely consequences of their actions. That's it. I don't want obedience.

Pa Pa explained his being a martinet by posing the question, "What if when your wife was five she was standing in the street and I saw a car coming and told her to run to me and she disobeyed?" I acted as if I had not heard him, but with you, dear reader, I'll share that I think such would not be as dangerous as for her to grow up not caring about herself or having wise judgment.

One night just before my eldest graduated from high school, I received a phone call from the mother of one of his friends asking to speak to her son. I expressed confusion. My three children were at home but no one else. She got quite agitated immediately, realizing her son had lied to her when he had told her he was spending the night with John Schroeder. I told her something within earshot of my three that I wanted them, as well as her, to hear. She knew I was a medical doctor and, I guess, credited me with enough knowledge or wisdom to allow me to calm her a bit. What I told her was not to advise her one whit; it was to comfort her; it was to advise my three. I said I knew her son to have good judgment and that he cared what happened to himself. I added that I saw it as not being so terrible if a high school senior on occasion would disobey and lie about his whereabouts to his parents, but I had a pretty sure sense he'd be taking good care of himself while he was doing so. That was what was most important—more important than, as a seventeen-year-old, to be obedient.

Dave Jr. told me a generation ago he felt he could be dropped naked and penniless out of an airplane in a parachute anywhere in the world and would be able to take care of himself. He wasn't bragging; it was said as a thank you to me for the travel I supported and the travel gene he got from his great-great-grandfather, great-grandfather, grandfather, and me (the Schroeder line all the way back to Germany, 1826).

In her early twenties my daughter wanted to travel in Europe, and I gave her a trip—paid her entire way—when she agreed to travel alone to a country in which the locals did not speak English. I'm really happy about how all three of my kids turned out. That is not because of anything I did; it's who they are, but it didn't come from making them obedient.

Now a story that throws promise keeping, obedience, and being good all in the trash: it is a story that caused me great embarrassment until I gave up my obeisance to shame. Now I can tell it to show how right was Dr. Phillips to have labeled me as despicably good, how breaking a promise is not untoward, and how true it is that you don't want obedient children. As an extra, it is a quaint vignette of the mid to late 1940s, which to me is a memory from only a moment ago.

During the first half of the twentieth century, the Pike in Long Beach was the premier fun zone in Southern California. In 1930 the newly constructed Cyclone Racer claimed to be the largest and fastest roller coaster in the world. Long Beach was a major Navy base, and at the end of WWII, the Cyclone Racer also claimed the (dis)honor of being the cause of death of a few drunken sailors who disobeyed the rule to stay seated throughout the ride. In 1947 during one of my family's occasional visits to the Pike, my safety-obsessed mother stood me at the base of the wooden behemoth, told me that I was never to ride it, and extracted from me a promise I would not. Fast forward to 1959: on a Sunday morning during a family conversation about the events of the weekend, I mentioned my girlfriend du jour and I had spent the prior evening at the by then decrepit Long Beach Pike, and I was describing the nadir of the park's decline, which had transpired as the result of the rise of the great theme parks in Orange County. My mother immediately queried, "You didn't ride the roller coaster, did you?" To my, "Of course we did," she wailed, "But you promised!" I easily replied that a seventeen-year-old today was not bound by the promises a five-year-old made over a dozen years earlier. Nothing more was said, and I assumed it to have been forgotten.

Now, here's the part that caused my shame until the package of rebirth that saved me from embarrassment emerged in late middle age. As my mother was aging, in her pre-dementia twilight, she told me I had never in my life disappointed her—except for the time I had ridden the Cyclone Racer. Geez, I never want any kid to be that good!

27

Prostitutes Are More Trustworthy Than Clergymen

I USED TO THINK I WAS JUST so, so clever to shock or amuse people by saying I've known lots of honest prostitutes but have never met an honest clergyman. Rather than demeaning the clergy, the shock was admitting I knew lots of prostitutes. Before you think I'm more interesting than I am, let me hasten to add I've worked in charity clinics, homeless centers, and an AIDS hospice back in the 1980s. And, yes, I did find the prostitutes to be as trustworthy as any other population.

I've also made references to the clerics whom I have treated. I have found some to warrant special suspicion as to their motives. Many of them I came to love, nevertheless. The only ones for whom I found an enduring distaste were the double-doctored ethics professor whom you've already met and five that you'll meet anon.

What has this to do with a book on happiness? It's an easy to remember (with a bit of a smile) lesson that life is better if not enslaved by what we were originally taught, that we shouldn't listen to still, small voices in our heads, and that ingesting the fruit of the Tree of Knowledge is never undesirable.

A prostitute gets paid by you to do what you want them to do. Usually there is an agreed upon fee. The clergy live off your donations to teach you to think and act the way they want, including how to please God with your contributions to them.

In my leisure I heard a quip I just love, and I'll share it now. The back story is that a TV news special some time ago featured four clergymen who were closet atheists but continued to minister to Christian congregations. They were interviewed with brown paper bags covering their heads and their voices electronically disguised–all for good reason. They professed to be perfectly ethical to preach doctrines they did not believe. Their rationale was they were paid to do a job, and they did it just fine. They saw it as no different than a Chevy lover who gets a job selling Fords. Rather than describe themselves as being like car salesmen, however, they described themselves as being paid performers who, like actors, recited the lines they were paid to deliver. It did remind me of Nuremberg, 1946.

Like prostitutes, they take money for performing a service in which they do not believe, but their congregations and employers must not know this–hence the hoods. The difference I see is prostitutes do it honestly. Why is it a tax deduction to pay evangelists to muck with souls and a crime to pay escorts to fuck with holes?

OK, the quip: on a camping trip to Saline Valley hot springs in Death Valley National Park, friends and I encountered a man sharing the pool, with whom a conversation developed. He was a minister in a church that has tenets all the way up the ladder of absurd. In an effort to ingratiate himself with our group who clearly weren't buying some of what we knew to be its doctrines, he went on the same tacks as the four in the sacks: he didn't really believe it, but he was good at his job. At that point my mate, Mike sitting next to me in the hot water made the statement that ended the conversation when he quietly but firmly opined, "Then you went from being a fool to being a crook."

28

Religion Is Like Circumcision

THIS CHAPTER HAS NOTHING to do with religious practices involving circumcision. It has to do with BS done to children by adults who can't undo what they have done.

I have a friend, Garrett, whom I admire, love, and respect and from whom I have learned a lot of what I am writing, even though he was not a patient. He was one whom I hired to teach me, being my personal trainer at Laguna Health Club for fifteen years. He has joined the crusade against the American practice of circumcising male infants. He believes this is barbaric and on a par with female circumcision done in cultures we consider primitive. He was circumcised as a newborn and feels he was violated. He has a lovely penis, a tad smaller than some, but he sees it as scarred and mutilated.

I've had patients who were not circumcised and went through their development years embarrassed, some severely, because they were different than their peers. My friend meets that observation with the advice that they can have the surgery after they become adults and then be just the way they choose to be. There is also a not rare procedure circumcised men may undertake to regrow a prepuce which was previously detached. There might be some data to be mined that show children whose world is their peers are traumatized by being different than their fellows, whereas some males who become wise to the world, like Garrett, feel more violation at having been made "unnatural."

I see to cut or not to cut as an unsolvable issue here and now in America, but I also see it as trivial, even though I was one who went through childhood and adolescence inhibited by my belief that I was in some way shamefully unlike my peers.

In so many ways, we make decisions for our children in the earliest years over which they have no voice or vote. We decide whether they will negotiate the years in which they form themselves with or without a prepuce, a prejudice, a religion, a vaccination, a home-schooled education, ignorance, street smarts, or just a name they may grow up to hate. We debate all of these issues to the point of nausea—at least the ones that are in the op-ed press du jour, but the kids get no vote.

I'm trying to use this chapter to underscore that in all areas of life, we can't give our kids a blank slate for them to write on as they grow up. We foul them up before they know how to set the ringtones on their iPhones.

If you raise them in the city, you deny them the advantages of Montana. If you raise them in a natural world, you deny them the culture to be absorbed in Manhattan. If you move a lot with your career, you deny them a stable milieu. If you let them grow up in one house, they don't get an early acculturation to other social environments. If you circumcise your boy or you don't, take your child to catechism classes, let them grow up agnostic, teach them your politics, raise them with any sense of values, let them play football, pierce their ears, don't let them get a tattoo at fourteen, or give them a car at sixteen you are denying them the opposite experience, and you will be criticized by some, vilified by others, and praised by only those who agree with you. I haven't even started on what we do to our children by choosing their diets.

Children are not traumatized by having believed in the Tooth Fairy or Santa Claus because as they get older, to an age where those beliefs don't work, they are surrounded by peers who also don't believe those things. The world helps them grow out of those childish ideas. But the world in which the child is raised does not help them grow out of their beliefs and scars and limitations in all the stuff that we don't think to put on the list of what needs to be addressed.

In the opinion of this experienced psychiatrist, all of the above pales in comparison to there being nothing in the world to help them grow out of the terrible belief that they should be better than they are whenever something is amiss.

Teaching our daughters and sons they need not be better than they are, there is no right or wrong, they get to do whatever they want to live with the unknowable consequences of doing, and no one is at fault for anything is, in my opinion, far more important than whether or not the kid gets religion, is circumcised, gets a proper diet, or has a stable environment.

We rightfully curtail child molesters, argue over religion, take our kids to soccer and music lessons and cotillion, for god's sake, and campaign for political power to shape the future economy and government for the sake of the next generation, but we don't free them from the BS and the SOB. No matter how we raise them, they are going to be imprinted with something to obey or rebel against. The best we can do is learn for ourselves as adults how to be happier and mentally healthier and pass that on to the kids as best we can and as soon as we can after we've already done the damage.

29

Sport Fucking Is Safer Than Making Love

AS A CHILD I WAS TAUGHT, as were many of my patients, that sex as an adolescent—or even as an adult—was dangerous out of wedlock for several reasons. It was a given it could lead me to go to hell, destroy my character, spoil me for the person I might meet some day, cause a pregnancy, and—horrors—transmit a sexual disease that would bring eternal shame on ... well, shame on everything. By the time I was growing up, antibiotics were available to treat the known STDs, and AIDS wasn't around. So the big horror of an STD was the humiliation, "Oh, the shame of it all!" The big risk was pregnancy—and disgrace! Then with the advent of AIDS, we were back to the dark ages again of being physically destroyed because we had transgressed.

I do get that some of this wasn't all wrong. The effect of such teaching was not lost on many a young couple who were in love and virginal until marriage. The others had to be concerned with birth control and with the secrecy that our prudish society would propound, but if they could get past that, they thought the risks were negligible. Limiting sex to one's main squeeze reduced the risk of disease.

People—real people—also have sex for fun, even when they are not in love, but they often believe they are in love and deny that they are doing it for fun only. They think they are safe if they can avoid pregnancy and STDs. There are a lot of people who have sex for fun, but they seduce their intended with protestations of love, leaving hookups surprised when they get pregnant or sick or find themselves alone.

Well, there is a risk that is more important than all of the above ideas combined. Warning of this risk is the why of the title of this chapter. The more we restrict our sexual behavior out of the concerns mentioned in the paragraphs above and the more monogamous we are, the more we might fall in love with the person with whom we are sexually active. Here is danger. Nobody in their right mind really knows how to pick a mate, at least not until they have had a lot of living and a lot of experience. Otherwise, the marriages that last and the ones that don't are pretty much a matter of dumb luck.

The risk of STDs and pregnancy are pretty slim compared with the risk of falling in love with someone who will not make a good mate. Shopping for the right mate with whom to co-parent should not be based very much on with whom one has the best orgasms. This point is even more important than the concerns of the health department or the moralists, and it is not often made or considered adequately in our discussions about sex.

Sport fucking might be safer. As I said in the previous paragraphs, forming a relationship which will be a happy union is often luck, often requires more maturity than is present, and is not science or ever a sure thing. We do the best we can and are responsible for making the very best relationships that we can make. Bonding with whom we share orgasms is now thought to have a neurological basis; thinking we are in love is bound to make that stronger yet.

Family, friends, patients, and myself have all come to grief because of believing the old saws about being in love being part of sex. When the biology says, "SCREW," the screwer tends to believe—either before or after or during the event—that they love the screwee. It is much safer to admit that sex is fun but understand and accept that falling in lust with one whom one screws is not commonly a valid basis for future happiness.

I don't want to get a disease from someone just because I was horny. I don't want to cause a pregnancy just because I was horny. And I don't want to fall in love just because I was horny. I want to use equal caution to not get emotionally involved with someone just because the sex was good as I use to not get the STD or the pregnancy.

Many of my readers may well feel the advice I'm giving is a few decades out of date and we're all more sophisticated today than to need this caveat. I'm also aware everything I'm writing will be taken out of context by someone whose feathers I'm ruffling. But it was only a moment ago I retired; I know what patients are still bringing up in sessions, and I believe falling in love with the wrong person can cause immeasurable grief. In the age of increased opportunities for sexual behaviors and experimentations of all ilk, I find it more important than ever to repeat this warning in a book whose purpose is to teach happiness.

I want to be very clear that I am neither advocating nor condemning casual sex. What I am doing is getting on my soapbox and preaching about a danger that can come along with sex that I find to be understated and therefore worthy of mention. By the way, this danger can come even with marital, monogamous sex. Common is the case of people in bad, even dangerous, unions that ought to be dissolved who stay just because the sex is so good.

Anyone younger than old, very old, has the fantasy that the one they love will love them so much as to be willing to change. This is not the case. If I have the greatest sex with a manipulator, indeed I fall madly in love with the manipulator, I need to be very aware that the manipulator will never stop manipulating. No deceiver will ever love another enough to stop deceiving. No lazy person will love another enough to stop being lazy.

It always interested me as to how one could have an affair with a married person, marry that person after the resultant divorce, and then be surprised when they learn that their spouse is having an affair which leads to their divorce.

It would be safer to sport fuck with an unknown or undesirable than it would be to fall in love with anyone who has a quality one can't accept. No one is going to love another enough to change a character trait. Any specific, highlighted behavior might change, maybe for a while; character will not.

Until one's identity is fully formed–again, probably the day before one dies–it is almost impossible to sort out in one's mind what part of love is nothing more than a fantasy of reassurance. A revered and widely published rabbi told me his insecurity was such that it was impossible for him to even listen to music without wondering if he liked the music or if he just needed to see himself as one who liked it. How much more terrifying it is to know that my choice in a mate is far more about what will make me think what I want to think of me than it is about that which I can't even comprehend for many years to come.

"Women might be able to fake orgasms,
but men can fake whole relationships."

SHARON STONE

"Sex: in America an obsession.
In other parts of the world a fact."

MARLENE DIETRICH

30

Never Forgive–Never Forget

WE ARE ALL STUMBLING through life the best we can. We are all perfect examples of what we are. Period. Who am I to think it is my place, privilege, or priority to forgive anyone for being what they are? No one has done anything to me. They have just gone through life being what they are. If I'm going to forgive my neighbor for being obnoxious, shall I also forgive Franklin Roosevelt for contracting polio and the Beatles for being British?

I have no reason to judge another person any more than I have reason to judge Mt. Whitney. If I were struggling with the Donner party to get over the Sierras before the winter blizzard, it would never occur to me that the mountains are anything other than what they are. Should is not an issue. Even though I die of starvation and exposure, it would never occur to me to blame the mountains, no matter how much I might hate them. Should I be a survivor, then would I forgive them?

I am very aware that readers might not easily equate a mountain's characteristics with the personality of their obnoxious neighbor or of the rapist or murderer that occupies the daily headlines. I maintain an individual's personality, their IQ, their brain damage, or their yet undiscovered peculiarities are just as real as is the fact of how high is a mountain. Yes, it will take eons for the processes of geophysics to change the height of the mountain, and it may take only a second for a person to realize the result of their behavior. Nevertheless, the fact that a second ago they didn't know what they learned a second later and are blind to most of the implications of their quirks is as much a fact as is the angle of a cliff.

I assume no one owes it to me to be any different than they are. There is no reason for me to blame or forgive anyone. I would lock up a child molester not to punish the pedophile but to protect the children. The reason for executing Ted Bundy should not have been to punish him; it should have been done only to protect those people who would have been his future victims—or maybe to discourage other offenders. With data to argue that the latter doesn't work there was no reason to off him. Well, save that after becoming dead he couldn't escape from any prison. Forgive is written on the opposite end of a sick popsicle stick from blame or punish.

I am not interested in how dangerous people are treated from the perspective of any humanitarian interest in those who cause pain to others as much as I am interested in preventing the pain of the possible future victims. For that reason, I'm more interested in lessening society's preoccupation with good and bad and punishment.

On the other hand, what folly it is to forget what one knows about one's world. If what another is is dishonest, I must remember that person is dishonest. I mustn't forget there are dangerous people in the world, and we must adapt a social, legal system to protect those who would otherwise be victims. This is just as I might learn I live in a flood plain and build a dam to protect my farm. I need not forgive the last flood, and I better not forget it.

To paraphrase George Bush's previously cited verbal incompetence: fool me once and I must never forget that you are a deceiver. I don't have to get even with you unless I still believe the BS, have not been BA, and think you have demeaned my self-respect. Then I must effect an SOB and kill you so I can again respect myself. After being Born Again, I just go through life realizing you have deceived me, and never forgetting that, I do what I choose to do to protect myself and society from you.

Maybe someday you do something to me that is totally out of character for you. You apologize profusely; you want me to forgive and forget. I will be a happier person if I remember forever that your lapse did occur and may or may not happen again, but the risk of same is small, and as such, I continue to be a close and trusting friend, well 97.6 percent trusting. How condescending it would be to deign to forgive, how unwise to forget, but how totally out of touch with the Born Again concept it is to blame! Without blame there is no grudge.

31

Apologize a Lot, but Never Mean It

BY NOW YOU KNOW, of course, my view that one is never wrong, never is to blame, and never need apologize. Happiness is greatly served by accepting that you are a perfect example of you—you are without need to be better than you are at any given moment but always with the potential to become more of what you want to be in the next instant.

If I did something thoughtless or unkind at 10:03 a.m., I may be sad when I realize I have hurt someone, but I do not blame or shame myself that that is what I'd learned to do up until 10:03 this morning. Maybe I think what I did was out of line with what I had learned—but it wasn't. Maybe it was something I almost never do; then it was something I learned to do rarely. Maybe it was something I abhor and teach others to not do. But if I did it, something in me was running counter to what I was aware of having learned.

When I see what happened, I may have surprise and sadness of any degree from trivial to overwhelming grief. I may want to do something to help or comfort the victim of my behavior, but I do not need to have shame, blame, or guilt that this was as far advanced in life as I was at that moment. I may well make note to remind myself never to do it again after 10:03:01, but I need not feel apologetic that I am the work in progress that I am. If you feel I owe you an apology, I would not disagree with you. I'd just rephrase it that I am entirely sad, want to make what amends I can, and determine to grow into someone who won't do that again.

If I'm careless and knock you over into a gutter filled with muddy water, would you rather have me blithering on about how very sorry I am, or would you rather I do all I can to help you? That may include all I can do to make you feel less assaulted. But I maintain caring about you will be far more useful than chattering on about myself and my state of sorriness.

This chapter is not about duplicity. It is about language. As you've read earlier, if I hurt someone the tragedy is not that I am imperfect, it is that the other person is hurt. I will do what I can to make the other person whole, and I will learn from the experience to change something in my behavior so I don't hurt others so often. But the sorrow I feel for the other person and my motive to change and grow does not mean I need to debase myself. What if I hurt you intentionally? Well then, if I am sad about that, I will be motivated to not have that intention again. If I am not sad about it, then I wouldn't have rendered a sincere apology anyway.

This caring for the consequence rather than being preoccupied with my innocence or guilt is a difficult thing to do, may take years, and might take a lot of therapy, but it is a goal worth pursuing. I have had patients who have come to me for help while grieved and depressed over something they had done which had hurt another—the ultimate being those who had killed their own children. Even though this is unspeakably overwhelming, the goal is still to get them to grieve over the loss, not hate themselves for not being more than what they were.

The world is full of people who do not understand this. When someone is angry with me or when I have hurt someone, that is not the time for me to begin to teach my message of how to be happy by being Born Again. It may be time for me to demonstrate same but not to preach it. I do not want to highlight every scar or pimple on anyone's face, just as I'm not interested in exposing every misunderstanding or neurosis. I want to understand the need of the other person, not drown my concern for others beneath my need to teach. If I hurt someone, I will say what I know to be the hoped for or expected sentiment by that person.

What I'm espousing is a lot like speaking a language. I don't expect my milieu to know the vocabulary I use. A similar issue occurs if I'm among people who don't speak English. If I were hungry while traveling in rural eastern Canada, I would not expect that to be true to myself I must ask for bread instead of using the word the Québecois will understand. It is not dishonest for me to use the word *pain* in describing what I want—even if I am not requesting an intense sexual experience.

I know I want bread, but I use *pain* because that will be understood by the hearer to correctly communicate what I want to say. For the same reason, I apologize a lot and often because that is the language of the people in my milieu, and I don't consider it a violation of what I believe. I understand I'm saying what I mean in the terms closest to what my hearer will understand.

I do find it useful to just eliminate the word sorry from my vocabulary when I'm trying to practice being Born Again. Sorry can mean two very different things. It can mean sorrow or it can mean apology. A big help in reinforcing this is to use apologize if that is the language of the one to whom I'm expressing the sorrow but to use sadness to describe what I feel when talking to myself.

Decades ago a Dennis the Menace cartoon showed Mr. and Mrs. Mitchell dressed for a social visit as they were leaving the house. Dennis asks them where they are going and why. Mrs. Mitchell says Mr. Henry has died and they are going to visit Mrs. Henry and tell her how sorry they are. Dennis asks the obvious question: did they kill Mr. Henry? Dennis took it that sorry meant apologize, although his parents were using sorry to denote sadness.

One night in a San Francisco restaurant, I was vilified because I had asked two women who sat at an adjoining table for forty-eight minutes after receiving their check if they realized there were people waiting for over an hour for tables. When I was told I was the rudest person whom this woman had ever encountered I simply said, "I apologize." Her screaming stopped and she simply walked out of the restaurant, leaving her table for the next party in line. That simple apology got me exactly what I wanted. I had no need to teach a pig to sing by suggesting it was she who was the rude one. (An interesting aside is that their table was next occupied by a man and a woman who upset the man to the point that he threw a glassful of red wine into her face and down over her white dress. I never returned to that restaurant, although the food and service were phenomenal.)

Try it out. Sometime when you are out with a friend and some critic faults you, just apologize. Your friend will wonder why you were so calm and accommodating, and you will explain you simply don't give any power whatsoever to insults, and you wanted the offender to just be gone.

I am not advocating appeasement of one who threatens. I'm just advising that my own insecurities are not proper motivators of responses. Handling an external threat needs to be done with all the resources one has at one's disposal. Those include not giving a fig for what the other person thinks of me other than the actual management of the threat. If one doesn't have a weapon, one might use one's legs. If one's legs are outrun, one might use one's ability to bluff. Sometimes a simple apology will save one's ammunition, one's legs, one's time, or one's neck. If saying "I apologize" will get you want you want, use it. If it won't, don't. And if your best judgment gets you shot, hate the fact you got shot; don't blame yourself–you can't have known what you didn't foresee.

I have a similar practice when it comes to using the words good and bad, right and wrong. If I am working with a patient to get them past the ideas that go along with depression and anxiety, or if I'm trying to help spouses to stop fighting, I will pontificate my doctrine for those purposes. I don't talk this way in normal life. You will find in this book that I casually use those words. Hopefully, this will only be when I am meaning to label something as being what we would want or not want. But I'm not going to censor anyone's–not even my own–usage of the words such that conversation becomes nightmare. If I am trying to teach the proper grip for learning how to be happier, I will make those distinctions. But even when testifying in court, I try to speak the language that will be understood by the listeners for the purpose at hand, not for me to be teaching them my tenets of happiness and mental health.

32

You Aren't Grown Up until You Die

WHILE BEING SCHOOLED in psychotherapy, I was taught that anxious patients often will become more anxious in the early phases of therapy. This is attributed to the fact that anxious people are often trying to do everything right, and they may become very anxious about how well they are doing in learning to be non-anxious. It's no different than a man who is so caught up in maintaining an erection that he loses his erection.

As an adolescent there was an occasion during which I was very anxious, and my mother gave me a Miltown to help me sleep. I lay awake all night worrying about what the pill was going to do to me.

It is common that those who want to become happier by applying the mental tools I am presenting will often become unhappy with themselves when they think they have got it and later see that they hadn't gotten it at all.

The reason I have disclosed discoveries about myself, including ones made while writing this book, is not just because I'm an exhibitionist; it's more, I hope, because I want my readers to get it that they will never get it. That's the reason I made up the example of the woman in the taxi who forgets her French when the vehicle flips on that boulevard in Paris.

To be happy one must accept the nature of things and concentrate on what's good. The nature of things is that we never get it right, and the closest we ever get is on the day we die.

Happiness demands that when we think we err, we remember it is not a mistake to be only as grown up as we are, and we have another chance at competency in the next moment. In my seventy-five years there has never been a moment when I knew how to walk perfectly or even swallow perfectly. There are aspects of my neurological system that let me know further growth may not take place in my coordination, but I fervently believe that next year I will be kinder and happier than I am this year.

33

Shakespeare Was Wrong

SPOILER ALERT: THIS CHAPTER IS ONLY here to give you a mnemonic to use when someone accuses you of being something you wouldn't want to be. I am not actually taking issue with the Bard, but "to be or not to be" is just all wrong outside of Prince Hamlet's agonizing.

Said another way, the infant might logically ask, "What am I?" but the only thing relevant to the adult is "What do I do?" To anyone developed enough to read, what I do is of importance, what I am (verb "to be") is moot. My question of my actions is vital, of my existence is inane. Descartes may have had a need to worry about whether or not he must be, but he was wrong about other things, too.

Whether or not I am good or bad, am honest or dishonest, am fickle or loyal is irrelevant. What is relevant is whether or not I do help you, do rob you, do hurt you, do pick up my trash, do contribute to my society, do raise my children well, do deceive or take advantage of others, and do live with the consequences of paying my taxes, driving safely, and keeping my brother. That is what matters.

I had a patient tell me his six-year-old was getting my message through him better than he was getting it himself. He was berating himself for spending too much money on a pre-digital SLR camera and then allowing his daughter to take pictures of the Grand Canyon from a lookout point. As the camera was doing that descent all cameras do when tiny hands hold them at the edge of a precipice, he began screaming at the kid because he was on that SOB of not being able to face his own shame when there was the option of blaming the child. But he was one of those fluid ones where the balance could tip back and forth as he blurted out, "What an idiot I am [verb to be]!" The girl looked up and said, "Daddy, what do you want to do [verb to do] about the camera being at the bottom of the cliff?"

I can appreciate negating Shakespeare is nothing more than a word game, and many think me pretty useless for pretending to write something that matters and framing it all in silliness. I admit happily what I am accused of is so, but look what this inane nonsense can do for one who uses it, as suggested, as a simple reminder of a usually forgotten aspect of being Born Again.

Morita was preoccupied with being helpless. Michael saved his ass by doing a face dive.

Dave Jr. related to me that he was called before his bosses and accused by a colleague of having been dishonest. In the midst of a vitriolic diatribe, David sat back and looked at options and decided what he wanted to do. Whether or not he was [verb to be] what the accuser alleged was never addressed by him. It happened that he had clear and simple evidence at hand of the wrongfulness of the allegation. But what he wanted to do was to express his sadness for all the angst that had come to everyone in the room from the advancement of a falsehood the accuser claimed to believe. He presented unambiguous documentation resolving the issue almost as an aside, placing his emphasis on decreasing the tension rather than making the malevolence of the accuser any part of the conversation.

Now, I do understand David has confidence skills that are pretty astonishing. The bosses present were in awe of his lack of defensiveness, and he was soon given a promotion and a raise. All of this doesn't come from carrying an overwritten Shakespeare around in one's pocket. That doesn't detract from the fact his response arose from his thinking that whether or not he was what the attacker claimed had to be back burnered to the issue of what he wanted to do (how he wanted to act) during the confrontation.

I am aware that an anecdote doesn't prove a case, but I had experience with so many patients for whom this concept was helpful that I deem it worthwhile to pass it along.

In a lot of crossword puzzles is found a clue of "Playground retort." The answer is usually "Am too" or "Am not." How very appropriate for the sandbox set.

34

The Golden Rule Versus The Diamond Rule

MERCY, MERCY! WHAT IS COMING next? First I attack the Bard for Hamlet's soliloquy; now I'm one-upping the Golden Rule.

I warned you I'd say things that only work in special ways just to get your attention and to help you hang on to a concept that might otherwise be forgotten. That's what I'm doing in this chapter and in the one above.

"Do unto others as you would that they . . ." As you would? How about doing unto others as they would want to be treated—not as you would want to be treated.

I happen to get aroused by pain during sex. That does not give me the right to bite the nipples of my playmate as hard as I might like to have mine bitten. I like to sit closer up front than most people at the theater. That doesn't mean if I'm taking you out to a movie I should subject you to my favorite seat. When I throw a party, I'm always unready at the appointed time and am glad when the first guest arrives only after I've remembered to sweep the herds of dust buffaloes under the sofa. That doesn't mean I should show up late for your invitations.

I'm certainly not trying to one-up scripture; as a rule for the masses this one has passed muster forever. But I like having a phrase to haunt me, to stick out, to remind me to care about another person, not to just care that I am a carer.

I can go around treating other people the way I want to be treated and never get to know them or how they want to be treated. The Golden Rule is a great one to teach, and I agree that I should show another the kindness and respect which I would want. But if I want to be happier than most and I'm willing to go back to the beginning and learn to think anew, I can do better. On every occasion that I take the time to understand another person, I am glad I did. If I make it my goal to know someone, care for them enough to want them to be happier, and treat them in the way they want, I'm happier.

I am a hugger. When I meet someone with whom there are positive feelings, I like to hug them. Shaking hands is for people with whom I want to perform the ritual of showing I don't have a dagger up my sleeve. Recently an event demonstrated the value of my Diamond Rule over the Golden Rule.

Among a group of relatives in my home was a handsome, young man whom I had met only once before. I enjoyed his presence as he was bright, intelligent, and just starting into a marriage and career—all things that make great subjects for conversation. Another guest confided to me that this man was homophobic, probably on the basis of some religious pretense. That was of interest only in that I then knew something about him that I didn't know before the confidence. When we were parting, everybody else got a warm hug, including his wife. But in saying goodbye to him, I chose to shake his hand while telling him how much I had enjoyed spending time and getting to know him. This goodbye did not occur in the midst of the group, so it was obvious to no one that I was treating him differently. The point was while I would have wanted a hug from him, I believed he would not want a hug from me. I knew something about him, cared about him, and respected his feelings and did what I thought he would have wanted me to do, rather than what I would have wanted done to me. Now, whether I was correct or not, I thought everyone else in the party was comfortable with being hugged by an aged homosexual. I believed he would rather have had a handshake.

I am not denying that this is what the Golden Rule teaches. I'm only using my Diamond

Rule as a way of reminding me to think again about the other before I just go doing what I would want.

I love the *New Yorker* for their cartoons which speak uncomfortable truths in a way that avoids the hostility of those too ignorant to get them. My choice for this chapter depicted two heterosexual couples in a Hamptons hot tub sipping bubbly in tall flutes. It was published in reference to ISIS-ilk terrorists. The stereotype is waxing unknowingly idiotic as she says, "I'm sure they'd like us if they got to know us." I'm sure her halo would shine like a score of suns were she to treat them the way she'd like to be treated. I'm also pretty sure there are no militant fundamentalists who would like it were she to strip them naked, dunk them in roiling hot water, and pour alcohol down their throats.

Last week I had lunch with Bob Simon. Bob is a physician colleague whom I respect and love above all others. I have never known him to be unkind. He never knowingly passed up a chance to comfort or to benefit another. I believe that he never did a medical procedure for the purpose of collecting a fee and never omitted a procedure which he thought would help a patient regardless of any probability of payment. His judgment is clearly better than mine. During our meal I ran the idea of my Diamond Rule past him—totally selfishly because I knew that he'd have something of value to add. He averred that the Golden Rule wasn't so trite as to deal with the farce of bitten nipples; it touted giving the consideration, respect, value, and concern to others that everyman personally wants.

I came home from that lunch realizing I hadn't yet conveyed the importance I was putting on my silly mnemonic. I agreed with everything Bob had said, but I still wasn't willing to ditch this chapter or its title. Remembering that line had been of too much serious help to me on too many occasions. Then I remembered when I had started using it. Again, it was a patient who was paying me to teach him who had taught me.

I had been working with a twenty-nine-year-old man whom I believe to have suffered more than perhaps any other of my patients. There was a too-long stretch of therapy in which he wasn't seeming to benefit from anything I could devise. That ended one day when he asked me what I was trying to do in response to a comment I had made. I told him I was trying to help him. His comment floored me when he said, "I would rather die than be helped. I want to be understood." I completely changed my approach, and the stagnation in his therapy changed into progress.

Remembering to not just treat others the way we want to be treated without understanding them is of everyday use when dealing with disabled friends who don't want to be fussed over and would rather do it themselves than be aided. It's useful in dealing with emerging adults who would rather struggle financially than have parents give them everything. It's terribly hard, but most valuable, when one is being left by a lover and is wanting to keep reaching out to the departing object of one's affection or lust, making a breakup lengthy that could otherwise be quick. (There was the boy who wanted to dock his puppy's tail without hurting the dog so much, so he cut it off one inch at a time.)

Perhaps the most common and important application of the Diamond Rule bears upon how we treat our children. To all that we say about loving our children and not making them wrong, we need to add that children must be respected. Too few parents will protect their children from the overly affectionate cuddling doled out by Aunt Edna, from the amusement that adult friends might find in the physical changes of a child in puberty, or from the over protectiveness of their own attempts to correct a slight suffered by a child who would, nevertheless, prefer that it be dropped. The second season of the television series *American Crime* deals with a high school student who is clearly wronged but begs his mother to drop her pursuit of justice—and the catastrophe which results from her pursuing her agenda for the sake of her son.

Of course, the most universal violation of respect for the child comes when a parent shows the affection the parent wants with no consideration of what the child wants in front of their friends. The same failure to observe the Diamond Rule has led some parents to shower things on their children without seeing that the child is mortified in front of his peers to have such things. Emily Post said back in the Roosevelt era that the only proper way to dress a child was in exactly what their peers were wearing. I've seen adolescents who were pained when the only option they had for transportation was to drive the car given them by parents who needed the child to drive a status symbol far beyond what the child wanted or was willing to be seen in.

There comes a time when the refusal of a parent to hand over to the child the next package of adulthood is more about not respecting the child than it is about over protectiveness.

This chapter even helps in caring for a pet. I recently got a new puppy (which I absolutely adore) and would want nothing but to be kind to the dog. I took it to puppy school expecting to learn how to train the dog, but I sat in jaw-gaping awe as Ryan had my puppy doing what he wanted the dog to do without any training whatsoever, just because he understood the dog.

"You have not lived today until you've done something for someone who can never repay you."

JOHN BUNYAN

END OF PART TWO

Lucile's Gospel

LUCILE KNEW how to be happy, and she knew how to be angry. She wasn't out to preach this, but her life did teach me almost all of what I taught. I'm determined her version of joy isn't going to die with her. I'm irked at the mendacity we all believe, so I will write. I'm doing this so what Lucile taught me about happiness won't die with me either.

My parents did not know this stuff. I can't blame them for teaching me the BS we all believe any more than I can blame them for the fact I only have two hands, but I am angry about it. Psychiatrists know better, but they usually explain the causes of unhappiness in a way that the gist of it doesn't get conveyed. The tragedy is so few in Western culture know the real joy of life, and those who set policy in our society maintain the myths that keep happiness elusive. It's a vicious cycle of the blind blinding the sighted before the latter have opened their eyes.

My mother was always drippy-sweet solicitous of Lucile but was forever finding fault. One day I asked her what it was she didn't like about Lucile. Her answer could have come straight from Tennessee Williams. She stammered, "She-she-she-she's always so HAPPY." She also could not stomach how elegant was the personage of Lucile. She absurdly attributed that to Lucile having married a man with more money than we had.

After they all had become dead, I learned the real reason for the antagonism. In the half decade before he had met my mother, my father was ensconced in academia at Berkeley and had carried on a correspondence with his cousin who was living with "the aunties" in Pasadena. He had never written letters like that to my mother. Lucile had saved Dad's letters; it's safe to say he doted on this cousin with an affection unexperienced by anyone else in his life. What my mother didn't know was the attraction my father felt for Lucile was not romantic or sexual but rather the attraction one feels to a happy person.

Happiness is a prosperity that one can experience even at the worst of moments. Lucile developed a temporary (although she didn't know it at the time) heart ailment and was bedridden alone at her home in Los Angeles. Her husband had just been placed in a skilled nursing facility, and she knew this new separation was permanent. I went to visit her with a handful of flowers. When I rang the doorbell she called out from the bedroom at the back of the house, "Come in; the door's unlocked. I'm in bed." As I entered her bedroom, she spotted the flowers and said, "Oh, that's wonderful. Put them in a vase on the dresser. When I look to the right I will see yours, when I look ahead I will see the flowers the neighbors brought me, and when I look to the left I'll see the birds building their nest in the tree just outside the window."

I had been close to Lucile for the then forty years of my life, but I had never seen her in any situation this bad. I didn't know how I'd find her. I said, "Lucile, you've got to teach me how to do this, how to have a life this joyful." She replied she'd always just been that way. She told of a time at age seven, living in the tiny Minnesota hamlet where she resided with her mother and "the aunties," when the entire town had gathered for the annual picnic—the ultimate social event of the year. Preparations had been ongoing for weeks. All faces turned dour as it started to rain—all faces except Lucile's when she blurted out, "Let's go inside and make fudge."

In one of the last years of her life during one of my very frequent visits to her, I was sitting in her living room after she had gone into the bathroom. She had not been well and was wearing a nightgown and robe although it was mid-afternoon. She called out that she needed me, and I went to find her. She had exploded with diarrhea and had liquid shit in her clothing, on the floor, on the walls, and—I'll never know how—on the ceiling. It became one of my most treasured memories of her as she instructed me on how to get her out of her nightie, clean her butt, get it out of her hair for god's sake, and mop up the room. What was so amazing, charming, and inspiring was the elegance and grace, which my mother had attributed to expensive clothing and accessories, did not diminish one iota under this most extreme circumstance. She was totally focused on what to do next with no cowing to the situation.

The part that made this all so valuable, so real, is Lucile knew how to grieve, to be sad, to be angry, to hate as well as she knew how to love and laugh. The amazing treasure of it all is she was a happy person when she was hating, grieving, sad, or angry. And she also knew how to boast to just the perfect degree.

For her ninetieth birthday I hosted the greatest party for her. It was held at my home in Laguna Beach and included the services of florists, caterers, hired musicians, and a photographer. I made sure no wedding could be a better celebration than was Lucile's ninetieth. I even found a comfortable chair for her! She gleefully rejected the car I was going to send for her and announced to me that she was driving to the party from her home in Los Angeles and was picking up two of her elderly friends along the way—picking them up because they, in their seventies, were "too old" to drive. The problem was Connie. Connie had been married to another cousin. When he had died, the family was just stuck with Connie. She was the most unpleasant person. Lucile had decided we would not invite her to the party because she'd introduce such a negative cast to the event. Then she changed her mind and said, "No, I want Connie there. All these people will be there to honor me and say good things about me, and I want Connie to see that!"

When she was ninety-three on my arrival for a visit she blurted out, "I'm just so angry," as I entered the door. I asked her, "Tell me." Her response was that she had just received the results of medical tests. She had been developing a neuropathy which was causing her to have constant pain in her feet. She lost her sense of equilibrium, she couldn't feel the floor, and she'd been falling, which she told me is scary to one in her nineties. The medical tests indicated the cause of the neuropathy was spinal stenosis, which doctors were not willing to surgically treat at her age. She told me she was going to have to live with this for the rest of her life. Her words were, "I'm just so, so very mad about this. Now, you have a new convertible, and I have a new haircut. Let's go for a ride."

After she became unable to walk, I was wheeling her to my car for an outing when she suddenly needed to urinate. There was no staff nearby, but there was a restroom. I pushed her into the room, lifted her onto the commode, and stood there holding my arm around her with her head on my chest and told her, "Lucile, we will get through this together." She and I were both completely clear I was telling her I'd be with her in her dying.

I asked Lucile later what she believed would happen to her after she died. Her response was, "Oh, I hadn't thought about it; that's none of my business. That's God's business." (I never did figure out which god she was referencing.) It was obvious that her being a happy individual had nothing to do with any belief about any place to which she was going.

When the moment came that she was to be no more, I was sitting on the edge of her bed. I thought her to be comatose as she had no signs of life except for a weak respiration and pulse. For whatever reason, I said to her, "Lucile, smile if you love me." She immediately moved every facial muscle into an exaggerated grin. She was clearly awake, and that was her very last communication. A smile!

Lucile understood to be able to hear the sweetest notes you had to have that same ability to hear gross farts; to be able to see great beauty you needed the same vision to see that which is ugly; to feel true happiness you had to have a sensitivity in your emotions which allowed you to feel great sadness. I saw Lucile in pain, in grief, while covered in shit, and when dying. I never saw her unhappy.

Lucile said she didn't know how she'd gotten this skill. Well, I don't know how she got it either, although the family tree reveals others on her branch to have been similar. There are so many theories of how it happens–biochemical, genetic, nurture/nature, and the crackpot beliefs that aren't the subject of any real thought at all. But Lucile did teach it to me–taught me how to be happy.

I pass on her "how to" often without even being aware. Patients frequently surprised me when they said when trying to apply what I had taught them in therapy they would ask themselves, "what would Lucile do?" I talk about her a lot.

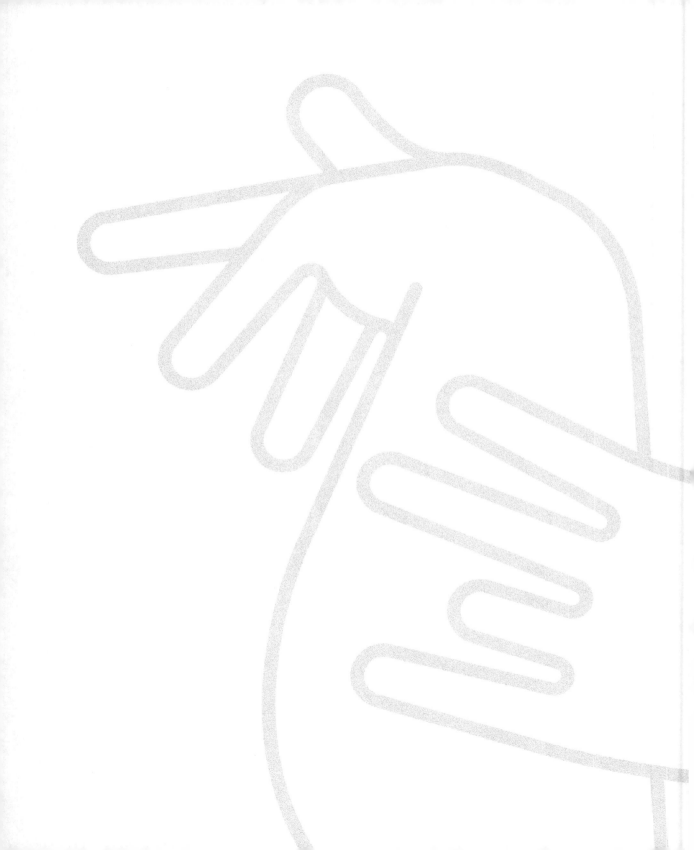

PART THREE

When You Know the Notes to Sing, You Can Sing Most Anything

In embracing emotions and actions as the thinking of infancy is replaced

by that of | *Born Again adulthood,* | *most of the causes of unhappiness just disappear.*

35

Love and Marriage

I AM PUTTING THIS CHAPTER FIRST in part 3 because it brings parts 1 and 2 together in a way that most easily makes these ideas practical. It is not the most important chapter, and there is no logical reason to put it first.

As a psychiatrist, I loved doing psychotherapy. I used medicine for those symptoms that medicine would alleviate, but I believed anyone could benefit from well-performed therapy just as any musician can learn to play an instrument more to their liking with lessons and any athlete can come closer to excelling with coaching or tutoring. Decades ago the media was embracing Dan O'Brien, whose Olympic gold medal in the decathlon in Atlanta designated him the number one athlete in the world. An article caught my attention that reported his work with two coaches in different states with whom he would regularly consult in his quest to yet improve. Clearly these men were not as good at performing as was Dan, but he did better with their coaching.

I insisted no one needed therapy any more than anyone needs athletic coaching or music lessons.

I told some of my patients they were mentally healthier than I, but I still thought coaching could help them to be happier. I saw therapy as being lessons in joy. After the insurance companies took over medicine and the ethics of business became the ethics of medicine, many psychiatrists altered their practices to concentrate on what would best be paid for by insurance. That did not include payment for physicians to talk to patients. I continued to do therapy and was told by one credible source that I was the last psychiatrist in the county to still do psychotherapy. Over the years, this reputation led many couples to come see me for what we called marital therapy.

The demographics of where and when I practiced provided me many such clients. For my first decade in practice I thought I was not good at it because I was trying to do what I'd been taught in training, and it didn't work all that well. I realized it wasn't me when my wife and I entered therapy with the most well-known and respected psychiatrist doing marriage therapy in the county, and what he did didn't work either. I came away from that experience thinking my wife was intolerable and he, at least to us, useless.

As I was learning from my patients the nuances I've tried to relate in parts 1 and 2, they spontaneously began to come out in the marriage therapy I was doing, and the results began to validate that approach. I came to see a simple pattern to what techniques worked and what did not. Basically, if one were to apply the ideas in part 2 about never believing in wrong and always taking responsibility without blame, marriages inevitably had a better chance of thriving.

There is a real chicken-and-the-egg dilemma in trying to teach this stuff. The first two parts of this book don't have much purpose until one reads part 3, and part 3 has no foundation until one reads parts 1 and 2. I can't fully grasp the importance or relevance of the theoretical stuff about BS and SOB and BA until I apply it to what causes the unhappiness in our lives, and I can't apply it until I understand the theoretical basis—even as it applies to Dillinger and Dahmer.

When the marital therapy I was doing became based on the absurdness of seeing anything as right or wrong, anyone as good or bad, any act as needing an apology, and there being no such thing as obligation, it began to be so effective that I came to be a believer in what I was doing and was able to apply it to my own divorce as well. I was able to be angry without blame, afraid without anxiety, and sad without depression. I was lucky to gain a reputation as being good at relaying to others what I had learned.

I don't have any data on this, but I would offer as a plausibility that if we married the person whom we love for what that person is, we'd have less divorces than in the current situation wherein so many marriages are based on loving the one that makes us feel good about ourselves. That doesn't guarantee a bad marriage, but it does mean we're selecting our mates on the basis of non-valid parameters. If I want a mate that primarily makes me look good and satisfies my sexual desires, I'm not choosing on the basis of finding one with a character with which I can live the rest of my life—or who will be able to live with me. It's like trying to get the best performing car by choosing the one with the brightest paint.

Competent marriage therapists are not trying to save all marriages. They are trying to turn what might be a bad marriage that could end in a bad divorce into either a good marriage or a good divorce. The therapist doesn't need to vote for which of the two will happen. If the couple stop seeing their positions as good or bad, stop being irresponsible, and stop blaming, either outcome will be improved.

To the best of my ability to remember, every couple who came to me on their way to a divorce lawyer consisted of two people each certain the other was wrong, each trying to convince the spouse that they were right, and each growing to hate the spouse for being unwilling to see what to them was obvious.

Back in part 2, I made some outrageous statements. By the time I came up with logical steps to make them true, it was also true those statements became inane and silly some of the time. Here is the reason for my having done that. How one treats one's spouse (and in later chapters, one's friends, children, employers, etc.) improves automatically if one just gives up any belief in right/wrong, good/bad, or blame. It's hard to convince a wife that her husband is not dismissing her value when she comes in crying that he didn't want sex with her, and then she espied him masturbating. It's easier if she already believes in not taking anything personally, if she doesn't believe in blame, and if she doesn't condemn him for having some sexual fantasies that don't involve her. The man who castigates his wife for buying a pair of Manolo Blahniks can be reasoned with if he understands that if he chose to marry a woman with this judgment and impulse control, a woman with this judgment and impulse control is what he gets. He may be presented with an unimaginable bill from Neiman's and with a perplexing dilemma, but his not knowing how to deal with this situation does not equate her with being bad.

I know this sounds absurd, but consider this. If I stop blaming my mate for what I do, stop blaming my mate for what they do, never make myself right or wrong, never make my mate right or wrong, I'm way ahead of the averages. Perhaps I'm married to someone to whom I should not be married. There are people who decide long into a marriage they'd rather be free than married. There are marriages ended by incompatible ethics. I've had husbands decide to become women, women decide they'd rather be married to a woman, and cheats who would rather be single so they can be promiscuous. In these situations, if the two could split with the smallest possible amount of animosity, that would be of benefit—especially if there were children. I would note that if blame were absent and if each took responsibility for their own behavior, the hatred would be less.

Intimacy becomes an essential part of any marriage that is going to survive. Intimacy is hard. It has different qualities than other human transactions, and it takes a long time to develop. It respects the other as much as it respects the self. It understands there is no right or wrong. It doesn't expect to hold together any marriage unless each party to the marriage wants the marriage more than they want to win whatever may be a conflict. It also means never giving in and never letting the self or the other be defeated; intimacy respects that one is not better—more right—than the other.

If a couple wants to enter marriage therapy, it is essential they find a therapist who truly understands the implications of intimacy and doesn't subscribe to the BS of right/wrong or good/bad. I cringe when I hear of troubled marriages that go into therapy with each party looking for a professional who will make them right or get the spouse to recant a position. I didn't say that correctly. Most couples who come for therapy start out that way. What makes me cringe is when they find a therapist who attempts to do that. A therapist who thinks their job is to be a referee doesn't understand intimacy.

If I saw a couple in which one party violated budgetary agreements and the other insisted on budget constraints, each would be insisting the other was wrong—overly stingy, selfish, dishonest, undisciplined, unreasonable, stupid, lazy, unproductive, ungiving, or worse. An argument would ensue, and each would begin to hate the spouse more each time they faced the issue. If I could use the concepts in part 2 and get each to see that the respective mate had every right to choose their own destiny, live as they chose, and face the consequences of their behavior, we would then have a chance. Maybe one would see that they would rather loosen up than be divorced, and the other might see they would rather cut back than live alone. But if they could get over seeing the other as wrong, then we had that chance.

One thing I saw over and over was if the two were trying to pull each other in opposite directions, there would be resistance. If there were no pull, they would often drift together. In an oversimplified way, let me explain it with a hypothetical: Woman who loves country music marries Man who only listens to classical. She tries to get Man to Stagecoach. He tries to get Woman to the opera. When he hears her listening to twangy, he insults. When she hears him enjoying a coloratura, she mocks. This is a single dimension used as a model. Of course, it is never this simple, but it often follows this pattern.

Let's change the scenario. Man feels it's just as important for Woman to enjoy Dolly as it is for him to enjoy Kiri. He turns down the volume of his music when she comes home. She does the same for him. She goes to Stagecoach with her girlfriends. He buys one season ticket for the San Francisco Opera instead of two. Over time, occasions pop up when out of curiosity—or just to be with the woman he loves—he watches the CMA awards with her on TV; she later enters a contest and wins two ballet tickets and goes with her husband. Over the years, Woman starts to enjoy Papa Haydn and Man comes to tolerate Hank Williams. OK, the music analogy was way too simple, but imagine a myriad of issues being handled in a marriage with no one being insulted or made wrong.

An aging gay couple told me the things they didn't like in their mates became endearing traits after the first fifteen years because of exactly this kind of respect and acceptance they had for each other. The next thirty-five years were bliss for both of them.

Nick and Nora each consulted an attorney preparing to divorce. Both of the attorneys, quite marvelously, recommended they see a marriage therapist at least once before proceeding with the filing. They came to my office not open to having the relationship saved.

I asked them why they were divorcing, and they agreed it was because they fought so constantly that they had come to hate each other and wanted out. I asked them to give me an example of one of their fights. The following was clearly not the basis for the divorce action; it is only one example of a multitude of arguments, but they averred it was typical.

Nora wanted to sleep with the window closed—it opened onto an area which she felt was not secure. Nick wanted fresh air. She wanted to sleep warm; he wanted to sleep cool. He thought her silly to worry about security. They lived in Irvine! She thought him selfish to value his comfort over hers. She wanted Asta in bed with her; he didn't want to be near the dog. He had begun to see Nora as doting, on the way to becoming decrepit. She saw him as cruel. They displayed, then and there in my office, a mien that would make me want to divorce either of them.

Nora scowled when I suggested Nick had every right to sleep in a room with fresh air and a temperature he found restful—and Nick smirked. They traded facial expressions when I then added that Nora had every right to feel safe in her own bedroom and to be snuggly and warm. Neither had wanted to sleep apart, and I agreed each had the right to sleep with their mate. My only intervention at this point was to maintain that neither was wrong, blamable, or should compromise. With that they demanded to know what I had in mind as a solution. I said, "Well, time is up; we'll have to discuss that in the next session." They walked out of my office united in an opinion for the first time, probably since their wedding day—the opinion that I was "a ass."

They returned for the next session with both wanting to work on another issue. I asked them about the bedroom and learned that was resolved; they wanted to move on to the next crisis. I stopped them and said if I were going to work with them, I would need to know how they had resolved the issue of the bedroom. They had bought a decorative security grill for the window, an electric blanket with dual controls, and a fan to blow air toward his side of the bed. They had spent $800, but they saw what could happen when no one is wrong.

I spent much effort a few chapters above trying to make understandable my claim no one was ever wrong. Nick and Nora just demonstrated why I went to the trouble.

By the way, Nick and Nora did not compromise. Compromise was Chamberlain and Hitler at Munich; compromise is what you do with the car seller when you're apart on the price. What Nick and Nora did was to stop making each other wrong. That's entirely something different. Each did what they most wanted to do, once they really understood each other. I'm aware that I'm opening myself up to an argument over my definition, which I could not win. Don't go there. I'm using this to plead that one stop making one's mate wrong and figure out what one wants to do when married to the person to whom one is married—that person having the right to be what they are.

I can remember many couples with whom I'd notice in the first moments of a session their standard operating procedure was to try to get what they wanted by making the other wrong. I would point out to them they were doing this, and they'd stare in disbelief. They had no idea of any alternative when there was a difference of opinion. My observation seemed as beyond obvious and unhelpful to them as if I were pointing out to them that they drink when they are thirsty.

I remember I only had a few sessions with Nora and Nick, and I don't remember—probably never knew—whether or not they divorced. They were getting along better when I last saw them. I don't brag about this being an example of any skill of mine—remember, they just thought of me as a donkey. I do, however, think it a good model for the changes that can come about if one stops believing the BS about right and wrong or the desire to make the SOB subject blamable.

Lucy needed to run into a store to return an item and thought it wouldn't take as long as five minutes. Ricky was going to wait in the car at the curb—in a fire lane—while she did it. They were on their way to dinner and a movie to celebrate their fifth anniversary. Lucy returned to find Ricky and the car gone. She assumed a security guard had told Ricky to move the car and he was probably making a loop around the mall. After standing there for about seven minutes, she noticed a fin of their '59 Chevy protruding from the stable of cars parked in an aisle a few yards away. Ricky was an idiot for moving the car and then not watching for her. Lucy was stupid and blind for not noticing the car when she first emerged from the store. I stopped them and led them on an exercise of how it would have been handled if neither had made the other wrong—if neither had blamed. Then what would have happened? They quickly came to see the evening would have been saved. As it had been, they abandoned their plans and went home not speaking to each other until our session, which was thankfully only two days hence.

If she had been able to tell Rick that she was angry without implying—and without him taking it as—he was wrong and if he'd been able to tell Lucy that he had gotten tired of waiting in the same vein, they could have comforted each other, learned something, and had an evening closer to each other than they were before the incident. Tragically, each was caught in the BS/SOB that says if one's mate is angry then one must make the mate wrong to preserve one's own self-esteem.

My favorite story about the benefits of taking responsibility for oneself arose when Jill came to see me about her unhappy marriage. (I never met Jack.) The tip of the iceberg was Jack would go to a bar with his buddies on the way home from work and get home after dinner was cold or ruined and Jill was in a state to nag and trash Jack. Jack would often apologize, which Jill came to totally disrespect, but sometimes he'd fly into a rage.

I told Jill that Jack had the right to come home from work any time he pleased, and it was up to her to figure out how she wanted to make herself happy while married to a man who came home a few hours after he had left work. She was quite upset with me for not helping her devise a way to make Jack more responsive to her needs, but she finally agreed to try what she saw as my plan. She came back two weeks later quite satisfied that my plan had failed because it had no effect on Jack's actions. We reviewed the suggestions I had made the session before, and I stressed that the goal had been to help her have a better experience while married to this man who Jack was. The purpose was never to change Jack's behavior; it was to make Jill a happier person.

She returned two weeks later with a tale I found not at all amazing. For the first week she actually started to have fun. One night she went to a movie and left Jack a note telling him she'd be back about ten p.m. Another night she fixed herself a meal about six p.m. and there were left overs Jack could reheat when he got home at eight. Another night she really wasn't hungry, so she went to the grocery, rented and watched a movie, and then fixed steaks for Jack and herself when he got home at eight thirty. The second week he was home every night at five thirty. On Friday he'd even taken the day off from work to go along while she was touring an old school friend visiting from Massachusetts around Los Angeles. When Jack came home at night and found his wife happy and having fun, he wanted to come home and have fun with her rather than spending time at the bar bitching about what a bitch she was when he came home late every night.

When I was a history major in college, I used to chide that the problem with learning from history is you never know what you learned. The takeaway lesson from WWI is jumping into action when diplomacy might work can be tragic. The takeaway from WWII is using diplomacy when jumping into action is needed can be disastrous.

Marriage therapy can be like that. In Jack and Jill's case, she needed to just shut up and take care of herself instead of going on and on about Jack not meeting her needs. Mary and Joseph were an example of exactly the opposite.

Mary came in alone complaining Joe never made her feel he loved her. She let him know she was unhappy. It didn't get her anywhere. I asked to see Joe alone before her second session. He told me he was frustrated because nothing he did would convince Mary of his love for her. He took time off from work once a week to have her join him for a restaurant lunch; he sent her flowers frequently; they had date nights often; they had sex 2.6 times per week and he would take all the time she wanted; he would call her from work every morning and every afternoon to see if she were having a good day. He had never been unfaithful, not even to the point of eying other women when he was with Mary. He didn't know what else he could do to show Mary how much he truly did love her.

Mary returned for her therapy session the next day. I shared with her my confusion as she verified every thing Joe had told me, including how often he told her he loved her. I asked her again why she felt unloved and her response floored me. Joe would rifle through the mail in the box every day when he came home before he would go into the house to greet Mary. Mary didn't think he would do this if he truly loved her. I asked if she'd ever mentioned this specific to Joe. Her response was, "What good would it be if I have to tell him?"

It's not just that Mary would not tell Joe or that Jill told Jack too much. It's that Mary wasn't communicating and Jill was nagging. Here's the difference. If you're telling your mate something they don't know, that's good communication. If you are telling them something they already know to get them to do something they have decided not to do, that's nagging. Communicate, don't nag. If you are sure that your mate knows what you want, drop it. If they choose to not do what you want, you choose to do what will not make the situation worse by doing it yourself or living with it not being done. Then realize you have a mate with a trait you don't like. Be angry without blame. A mate has the right to determine their own actions. You get to decide how to make yourself happy while married to this mate. Maybe you make yourself happy by shooting your spouse, seeing a divorce attorney, fucking their best friend, or by seeing what will happen if they know you make yourself happy even when you don't get everything you want. You get to do whatever it is you think will yield you the consequences with which you wish to live, but you do it understanding of the consequences of nagging.

The male/female roles could have just as easily been the other way around in the above case histories. This is not a sexist issue. These examples came to mind because more often a woman will come asking for help than will a man. Whoever asks for help is the one who is the focus of the therapy. In gay couples, both lesbian and male, it is exactly the same.

If one communicates with one's mate what one wants and then goes about making oneself happy with what one gets, marriages tend to be better than if one doesn't communicate or sets out by any means to get the mate to do what the mate doesn't want to do. All of these suggestions arise from the understandings theorized in part 2.

Forget the Bullshit of believing something is wrong with you if you don't get what you want, and don't make a Shift of Blame to accuse the other instead of blaming yourself. The Born Again response is that nothing is wrong with you and nothing is wrong with your mate. There is no blame. Go after what you want, and what you don't get you live without. It's your responsibility to make yourself happy in or out of the marriage.

If alcohol, incest, promiscuity, financial dishonesty, or murder are involved, it doesn't change the above one whit; I can say that from experience, having dealt with all of that and more. You are being irresponsible to stay in an untenable marriage and try to make your mate be a different person than they are. If you can live with it, make yourself happy and do so. If you can't, get out.

When victims of domestic abuse stay with the abuser in hopes of being able to change the abuser, they are unconsciously holding on to a remnant of infantile omnipotence, believing in their power to influence what is in fact a quality outside of themselves over which they have no influence.

Sam and Delia came to see me at Sam's insistence because he wanted to save his marriage. On entering my room, before even sitting, Delia was on a rampage the likes of which I'd never seen before or since. She raged on for sixty minutes; I would swear she never even paused to take a breath. Can one breathe without a pause? Neither Sam nor I had uttered a syllable. We had exceeded the session time limit, gone through what would have been my piss and coffee break, and I had another patient in the waiting room. I wanted them out of the office, hoped we could continue in another session, and tried to segue into an exit. I got only as much said as, "Delia, I can see...," at which she jumped up, accused me of taking Sam's side like everyone else, and fled the room. Sam told me this was his last attempt at trying to save his marriage. No previous attempt at therapy had helped. She had, during past fights, actually tried to kill him on three occasions. I endorsed Sam's plan to stop trying to save his marriage. I'd still argue that happiness for Sam would be enhanced if he could acknowledge that Delia is what Delia is and the question is what is Sam going to do.

I have seen patients who did not stay in treatment and who later attempted to murder or did murder the spouse.

I've just explained how I would utilize the concept of not blaming to save what could be saved in relationships. To make it simple, I'd say if you marry a person, that person is what you get. If one marries a man who stinks, that doesn't obligate the man to stink less. Maybe the mate promised to use deodorant and now won't. Well, if I marry one who makes promises to be unfulfilled, then I married a stinker who doesn't do what they say. One doesn't obligate the other to do what was originally planned. If we both promise to honor and now that mate disses me, then I have to make up my mind what I want to do about being married to a ball-breaker. The relationship can't be saved by threats, blame, or an SOB. I would need to accept that my mate is a disser and realize it is a trait of a mate who is in Group B some of the time. My mate has the right to be in Group B, and we just need to find a way to cope with it or split. Maybe some way to shock the mate into an insight would work, maybe a more honest conversation of how much it hurts, maybe learning to not be hurt, maybe some application of a combination of styles mentioned in earlier paragraphs.

My favorite story was of a woman who dropped by the house in the midst of a workday and found her husband in gravity-defying positions with the pool man. Her response was to jump right in and make it a three-way. That they failed to notice her presence presaged their divorce. That came from Steve Schalchlin and Jim Brochu's musical *The Last Session*, easily as good an experience as I've ever encountered in a theater.

I still believe in marriage therapy. It's easy to just tell someone to stop blaming their spouse and make themselves happy, to communicate but not nag, to realize you want a good marriage more than you want to win an argument, and giving in will always come back to hurt the marriage later. Telling them just gives encouragement. It's only marginally better than yelling at your girlfriend to hit the ball. But if over time one can get the parties in a marriage to be healthy in expressing their anger without blame, acknowledge there is no right or wrong or good or bad, learn to experience joy and sadness without pride and shame, not wait for time to heal rifts, etc., then a therapist can do better than a motivator who just yells "Fuck yes" repeatedly to punctuate encouragement.

If Olympic athletes still learn from coaches, prima ballerinas still go to dance class, and professional musicians still benefit from critics, one can be sure a therapist who understands how to teach others to dump the BS and avoid the SOBs can help marriages toward either thriving or ending without devastation.

"Winston, if you were my husband,
I'd poison your tea."

LADY NANCY ASTOR

"Nancy, if I were your husband,
I'd drink it."

WINSTON CHURCHILL

36

I Am . . . I Said

THE ATTITUDE I WANT to describe now is never completely attainable—at least not for anyone I've ever known, except maybe in my idealized visage of Lucile. The more I focus on trying to reach a point, the more happy I become. That point is zero. I want to see myself as not a positive or a negative. I don't want self-esteem, and I surely don't want self-abasement. There is no question as to whether or not I am. "To be or not to be" is of no importance—it's just not an issue. All the questions in life are about what I want to do. I am not good or bad. There are no modifiers as to what I am. If I want the consequences of working, I work. I am not industrious or lazy. If I want all of the consequences of killing my neighbor, then I kill my neighbor. I am not good or bad.

I learn to hate the things I hate without making me right or them wrong. I can kill a rattlesnake if it threatens without making the rattlesnake bad or wrong, and I can fear the snake while I do it. I want to protect society from serial killers; it's not a roadblock to helpful behavior if I hate them while I do it. If I don't believe the BS about hating, then I have no urge to blame or punish even though I hate. I don't want to settle a score with anyone.

If someone is furious with me, I'm sad for their discomfort and also sad for any discomfort they may cause me. For that reason I try to not make people furious. I don't feel bad about me if someone challenges me, even if I am frightened by their challenge.

There is no amount of racism, misogyny, homophobia, xenophobia, self-righteousness, religious intolerance, greed, or jealousy that will cause any problem if the so infected realizes such is a neurotic trait from which they have not fully emerged and know it is not something to be acted upon. The more comfortable one is in seeing oneself as having such thoughts, the less likely it is that the thoughts will intrude into behavior.

Jimmy Carter looked on a lot of women with lust and committed adultery many times in his heart. No scandal or hurt came to anyone from the ideation of his libido or from his admission.

I would grieve so when a patient would tearfully, painfully confess to me (a priest I am not!) some thought, obsession, emotion, or ideation over which they felt shame or guilt. OK, we've dealt pretty thoroughly with the whole ridiculousness of shame/blame/guilt, but let's discuss some specific issues about thoughts and feelings.

Absolutely any combination of phrases or ideas or images the brain can produce it will. Dreams are a good example of how crazy our minds can be. My mind will come up with murder, perversion, depravity—well, anything of which there can be a thought. If one sees this as curious, interesting, or amazing not much ever comes of it. But as soon as one assumes they are a bad person for having such thoughts they get unhappy. The same can be said for the true emotions. Experiencing any degree of them does not change what I am, doesn't tilt my scales one way or the other.

In part 2, I covered the value of embracing sadness and grief but rejecting shame or guilt or blame, even (or especially) in those areas in which our milieus try to ameliorate grief. Here I want to discuss some specific examples of how this practice can make us happier with what roils our guts and what strangles our hearts.

At Christmastime 1972, I attended the funeral at Rose Hills Mortuary in Whittier, California, of a college student who was the son of a close colleague of mine. He had been killed in a car accident a few days before on arriving home from school for the holidays. I have never forgotten the nausea that swept through me when the minister admonished the audience we should not grieve that God had picked this rosebud for his garden in heaven. Irrespective of one's theology, dissing us for grieving was just obscene and about as ignorant as was his sense of horticulture. Clearly any hooker might have clearer, more truthful counsel. It would have been better to have made syrup out of that sap than to have listened to him.

Exactly seventeen years later I was in St. Patrick's Cathedral for the funeral mass of Billy Martin, who was also killed in a car crash at Christmas. I remember just as clearly Bishop Edwin Broderick's admonition that we should grieve greatly over the loss, because the grief was our testimony to how much we loved him. I can't say I loved him; I'm not enough of a Yankees fan to even know much about who he was, but the gulf between the New York bishop and the Whittier preacher man will never be forgotten.

Crying doesn't help. Suffering doesn't make you stronger. It just aches. But experiencing those emotions is like riding on a roller coaster. If you just let fly and flood yourself with the feelings, you go crashing to the bottom and rebound right back to mental health. If you put brakes on the hurt and try to avoid the pain, you just skid to the bottom and sit there.

You can stand any combination of pure emotions; what will make you sick mentally and physically is the perversion of those emotions that results from believing the BS that turns them into guilt, shame, pride, blame, anxiety, and depression.

Lucile focused on how very, very mad she was for a few moments and then was ready to go have fun.

A patient always feels better when their psychiatrist reaffirms a situation really is as painful as the patient perceives it to be. They feel better because someone voted for them having their feelings rather than against.

I will be sad. I will hate. I will fear. I will be lustful. I will want. Anything that makes me feel self-abasement because of those emotions will cause trouble that the sadness, hatred, fearfulness, desire, or want would not.

Being exposed to the horrid, slithering sound of a thumbnail scratching on a blackboard will make me hate the noise, but it does not make me want to be deaf. Seeing an image of the cruelest ugliness won't make me desire blindness. How strange then that people are afraid to love for fear of abandonment, to trust for fear of being made a fool, to give for fear of being exsanguinated.

I have learned from patients who have lived the most extreme grief, fear, and anger—far more than have I or anyone in my personal life experienced. What I have learned from them, I have passed on to others subsequently. I give that first quadriplegic patient credit for what he taught me that I was able to pass on to the others I encountered that same summer. Patients have taught me no matter how extreme the pain, there is a maneuverable component to how much one suffers.

My friend and physical trainer, Garrett, taught me I don't have to abort a repetition because of intense pain. The need to stop the rep comes from the terror that the pain felt would increase in the next instant. But at the given instant, one could stand the pain and finish that rep. I have been in depressions in which I was able to isolate and see that a component of the depression was the dread of the next moment of depression. I've been able to stand depressions with just the knowledge they were temporary. It was not a matter of time curing them; it was a matter of feeling better right now because I knew I would not have such pain for long.

Before having better sense, I went through one depression in which I was able to continue to work and function through a six-week period in which I'd see a patient for fifty minutes, cry for ten minutes, see the next patient for fifty minutes, and then cry for the next ten. Amazingly, only one patient seemed to catch on to what was happening. The poorest functioning person I was seeing at the time said one day, "Doc, you don't look so good!"

When I got better sense, and when safer and more effective drugs came on the market, I began taking Prozac, but that first time I got myself through by using my existential trick. There will be more about this in my next chapter. Basically, I kept concentrating on the reality that my brain chemistry had shut down; it would recover soon, and all I needed to do was hang on until it did. The thoughts of hopeless despair were delusions.

Just as bearable pain can become unbearable if mixed with shame or guilt, looking for the silver lining can tarnish one's pain. Hope can turn a nightmare into perdition. Unbearable pain can become bearable when the one in pain discards the shame/blame/guilt, rejects the power of positive thinking, and instead isolates out the pain itself knowing it is temporary, it is not deserved, and it does not lessen the value or potential of the self.

The best model for me when in sadness, grief, pain, anger, or fear is to imagine I'm standing with my nose touching the outside wall of a barn. The color red fills my entire world; there is nothing else I can see. Living through time is like slowly stepping back from the barn. There comes a time when the barn fills my entire world view, but I can begin to see edges of grass and sky peeping into the periphery. Later, it is huge, but I can see the rest of the field. Many more steps back and it's only the biggest thing there is, but there are a lot of other things in my vision, just not as big. After stepping back for a mile, I can still see the barn and it's still the same red, but it no longer prevents me seeing other things. If my vision is telescopic enough, that red barn will be in my perception for all of my life; when I do look at it, the sadness or grief or pain or anger or fear is still the same red. But I am also alive and can thrive. Accepting this model, I feel somewhat protected from devastation even on day one. Believing that I am devastated can cause decompensation that withstands all time.

I am stunned when I learn of one who survived Auschwitz or Dachau and later had any semblance of a life. I can't imagine it. I'm actually so old as to have had patients who'd been there. I've had patients who have suffered in other ways I likewise cannot imagine. They taught me that if I would just be there, holding their hearts with them, they'd also reclaim a life worth living. Trusting in that process of letting nothing change one's worth worked a bit, when hoping it was not as bad as it was or trying to find something good in the abyss would make it worse. But time won't work if one is still taking the grievous issues personally, blaming or shaming, or needing to punish.

"They also serve who only stand and wait."

JOHN MILTON

37

What'll I Do?

UNTIL ABOUT THE AGE of sixty (60!), I was awkward and unhappy with the way I behaved whenever someone paid me a compliment. I wouldn't bother to put this in a book except I came to learn this was a very common problem among those who were consulting me. After years of talking about Group A and Group B, it suddenly hit me I was being very insecure and had not applied to myself what I had been teaching. In spite of disseminating all of the above ideas, which I fervently believed, I was still blind to my own BS and was acting as if compliments were about me.

It seemed to me I was grandiose or else naive and gullible if I believed a compliment, so I would want to somehow weasel out of it and deny such kind words should refer to me. Suddenly, in one spurt of understanding it dawned on me to apply what I was teaching others to myself in this particular situation. The compliment was not about me; it was about the complimenter. My problem with compliments evaporated when I saw that my response should be about them, not me. How rude it had been of me for all those decades to discount the other person's opinion in the attempt to appear humble—or worse yet, to appear smarter than they in assessing my own inadequacies. Speaking even more to how blind I had been, I had applied my Group A/Group B solution to insults for years, but not to compliments. If someone had insulted me, I at least knew—even if I couldn't feel—that it merely spoke to the insulter's opinion. I was better at not being hurt by an affront than I was at not having pride at a compliment—pride which I defended against by denying the validity of the compliment.

The simple solution was to apply to a compliment what I been applying to insults. If I thought I had done a mediocre job and someone told me I had been great, I simply expressed my happiness they had found some joy in what I had done and thanked them for taking the time to tell me. I didn't respond on the basis of what I thought of me; I responded on the basis of what I thought of them. If I wanted to be more gracious, I'd elaborate on how I valued their sharing their perception, not on explaining anything about me or my performance. At that moment—to the extent I could actually do this—I was acting as an adult rather than acting on the basis of BS which would have said I was great if they thought so.

Earlier, back when I was still an idiot in my blindness to my own problem with this, I was able to use this principle to pull off a one-session cure for an anxious young man—well, a cure for one symptom anyway. His specific reason for consulting me was that he was too anxious to approach an attractive woman to ask for a date. He was paying me for my time, and I felt I owed it to him to send him out of the office with a solution to his problem that day. If he wanted to see me later for other issues, that would be fine, but I wasn't about to string him along into further expense and time by listening to him unfold his whole psyche while I passively would steer him toward finding his own solution. I knew a technique he wasn't using, and I was going to teach it to him that day—based on my rejection of BS.

I asked him if it were true that he would feel badly about himself if an invited woman rejected him—or worse yet, insulted while she rejected. He didn't understand why I would ask that as it was so obviously true. I then asked him if he'd feel better about himself if she accepted—or better, was thrilled he'd asked her. He agreed that both questions would merit a very strong yes, of course. I then explained the concept of Group A and Group B.

I told him to go home, stand in front of a mirror, and strip naked. While looking at himself in the glass, he was to consider his intelligence, his manners, his skin, his muscles, his genitals, his achievements, his body odor, the frequency of his farts, etc. For the sake of the argument and to err on the side of conservatism, we conceded that 61.3 percent of women would reject him—that which he was viewing in the mirror–and 38.7 percent would date him. I asked him if he were willing to go check out whether a given woman were in Group A or in Group B, guessing about three-fifths would be in Group B and two-fifths would be in Group A. Did he want to date attractive women enough to learn into which group any one of them would fit? He'd remember that naked assessment in the mirror and realize which group the woman was in was the only issue, and it should have no effect on what he thought of himself.

He returned a few weeks hence to tell me he'd asked six women out, four had accepted, and he'd had a lot of fun with two of them, one of whom he was planning to see again. He'd had no anxiety about any of the responses being good news or bad news about him, although he was excited with the prospect he'd finally get laid. During that appointment I did an assessment as to whether or not there were other symptoms, depression, suicidal ideation, or substance issues for which I might urge further treatment. He seemed really happy with his progress after only the two sessions. I urged him to try to apply what he'd learned to all aspects of his anxiety and to return only if he found he wanted to learn more. Now, I do realize that stage fright in all its variations has a basis in brain chemistry as well as in the way one thinks. Nevertheless, if I give up the BS that I have to think less of me if another thinks less of me, it helps.

If anger were causing behavioral problems, I'd urge the subject to get angry more often (that advice would make them angry!) and to desensitize themselves to being angry. We'd practice on the simplest of things first. I'd instruct a patient to amplify their anger when coming upon a red light. They were angry the light turned red. There was no one to blame. There was just a pure sense of not getting what one wanted. It was not a sign that they'd been driving too fast or too slow. It was not the fault of another driver who had impeded their speed. The patient would retort that my suggestion was inane; they didn't get angry at red lights. I'd explain the problem was that they'd only perceive anger when they could blame, and the need to strike out was actually only the need to not blame themselves by punishing another. Therapy was to get used to the idea of anger as meaning only they weren't getting their way, absent any blame or need to punish. They also had been aware of anger only when it reached a boiling point. A step in treatment was to experience anger as an emotion that occurs anytime one didn't get what one wanted, no matter how trivial. They protested that would be infantile and narcissistic. I explained how that perception was the problem. Because of this fear of being a baby, they'd not allow into consciousness any anger unless it was significant and the result of some tort done to them. Then, there would be a problem—no, a PROBLEM! If one can't know one is angry at a red light, accept the anger, and just stop the damn car with ease and tranquility, then how could one expect themselves to find a spouse in bed with a best friend and accept this anger and just find a new spouse and make a new best friend with relative ease and tranquility.

I agree the above paragraph sounds as if I'm an idiot, but I'm not stupid. Understanding one's anger and needing to do nothing about it at the red light is like gripping the racket. Not murdering your wife and ex-best friend is like winning multiple Grand Slams. But when one does not understand how to grip the racket, there is no point in going further in training for a championship. Until one can get angry and not see it as a sign of anything needing to be righted, one cannot move away from outbursts. Therapists who try to make patients learn to be less angry are on the wrong track. They need to get more angry more often but—silly as it seems—learn to be happy with their anger. We're right back to my first comments about cholera. The water is fine, the bacilli can kill you. The anger is fine, the blame or fear or shame can kill and often does. The blame and fear of shame are bigger in the case of the cuckold than is the anger or grief itself.

Existentialism is a great tool to use for the purpose of becoming happier with one's behavior. Unfortunately it can be difficult to learn and takes a lot of practice. Now, I'm the first to admit I don't even know what the modern French philosophers are about. But let me share with you the special application I use that makes for a simple understanding of what is.

Imagine yourself to be in a cinema watching a horror movie, and imagine your behavior for some reason isn't pleasing you. Maybe you're more terrified than is fun, maybe you're going to cry, maybe the last time this happened you pissed your pants, maybe you're just having such fear that you want to grab the stranger next to you. What I mean by existential is that you concentrate very hard on the fact you are in a theater; light images are flashing on a screen in front of you; electricity is making its magic in the Dolby sound system. Look up at the ceiling and all around you. See that you are sitting through the presentation of a movie; you are not in the movie or in the story. Or try judging whether or not the cast is competent or if the story is cohesive. When you get good at this through practice, you'll find that the terror subsides almost immediately.

Another application of this non-philosopher's use of the E term would happen when my young male patient, above, would concentrate very hard on his quest to learn if a particular woman is in Group A or Group B. That a woman has no power to judge him and has the power only to reveal what are her proclivities is what is. The cinema is what is. That the woman can really evaluate, that the horror on the screen can engulf is not what is. One who has no faith in their ability to cope can see the possibility of coping when the BS is removed and one is dealing with the essence of what is.

On the subject of one's own behavior, I want to throw in the story of Martin, a twenty-two-year-old man who was suicidally depressed. Friends had compelled him to come see me, but he saw no point in it. He knew there was no point in his living; his life would only come to ill, and he would become so depressed he would entertain suicidal ideas.

My assessment led me to believe he was not in immediate risk. His need was not protective confinement but longer-term resolution of his biological and psychological depression. All he was aware of was that he could not stop masturbating, and he believed from what he'd been taught by some church that he was condemned unless he would stop. I am not so naive as to believe that his inability to stop jerking off or his belief in it being a sin was responsible for his depression, but it was his presenting complaint. His concern with this issue had preyed on his mind since puberty, frustrated him, guilted him, and caused him to feel morose and devastated by any sexual interest.

Those pricks who taught him that he was anything other than healthy and normal for masturbating certainly harmed him as much as if they had sodomized him, fellated him, or stuck a cock down his throat.

He had never been physically molested, but his psychological damage was as great as if he had been. It has always saddened me that Martin never returned for a second session. He came once as his friends had implored him to do. He could now go back and tell them he was hopeless. He had come with a mind filled with "truth" and left with "truth" intact. Thankfully, few in our society any longer believe masturbation is untoward. For the large part, either they stopped believing the BS about playing with one's attached toys or they have come to see that their intimidation on that matter is pathologically passé.

To illustrate how social attitudes can effectively neutralize dogma, I love to tell a story from a friend in England. He is a gay man in his forties, happily married, and so emotionally together that he is trusted by the Catholic boys' grade school in which he teaches to conduct the sex education classes. I have visited his class of fifth graders and found the room to be filled with cherubs, each dressed in blazer, white shirt, and striped tie. He told me the first time he had broached the subject of masturbation in a sex education class, he expressed curiosity as to how the boys related to the fact the Catholic Church teaches self-amusement to be a sin. He described the purest, sweetest, most heart-meltingly angelic boy in his class raising his hand and, when called upon, proudly announcing, "We sin a lot, sir!"

Dealing with compliments, fear of approaching others, stage fright, anger, coping with fear, being late, getting things done, masturbation, and pornography are only a smattering of issues patients have brought to me concerning their dissatisfaction with their own behavior. What these things have in common is all are based on the infantile belief I'm not good enough unless I'm better than I am. The effect on the psyche of the BS is truly BS.

In the 1980s I attended a week-long continuing education course at Mt. Sinai Hospital in NYC. It consisted of lectures given by specialists in all other fields of medicine to keep psychiatrists abreast of what was going on in other disciplines since they had left general medicine to specialize in mental health. I remember the chest surgeon never mentioning smoking in his presentation. During the Q and A he was asked why. He reminded us that the orthopedic surgeon who had addressed us had not discussed whether or not falling from the eighty-sixth-floor observatory of the Empire State Building could be damaging to one's bones. He felt a discussion about smoking and chest ailments would equal that as an insult to the intelligence of his audience.

I choose to not extend this behavior discussion by going on to addiction issues. One's behavior regarding drugs, tobacco, alcohol, gambling, as well as a host of obsession problems is so well understood to be impaired, not helped, by guilt/shame/blame it would be an insult to my readers to even discuss that. And to write further about how the infantile application of Bullshit, Shift of Blame, and lack of rebirth contributes to racism, homophobia, bullying, xenophobia, and puritanism would belittle my readers as much as if I were to seriously lecture them about the relationship between smoking and cancer, between falling out of the sky and fractured bones.

38

Children

YOUR CHILDREN ARE NEVER wrong. Never. Never tell them they are wrong. Your children don't know what happens when they run into the street. There is nothing wrong with them in not knowing what happens when they run in the street. They are not aware of ethical issues, of what happens if they do or don't do as they are told. They don't know how to, or why they should, modify their impulses. That is not something wrong with them.

Virtually everything a parent wants to correct in a child is something that the child will grow out of on their own—screaming, running in the street, throwing food, torturing the cat, finger painting on the wall, setting fires, lying, disobeying... The parents need to keep the child safe, protect their property, prevent the behavior from blackmailing them, and refrain from making the child feel that the child is bad until the child grows out of the behavior. A very intelligent, sophisticated, worldly wise grandmother was listening to my ideas and wanted to know how to stop her grandchild who was throwing tantrums without making the child wrong. She was floored when I suggested that she simply comfort the child that the child can't have whatever it is over which they are throwing the tantrum. What would one suppose would be the consequence of a child learning a tantrum will get them nothing from a parent or grandparent who doesn't fault them and supports them in their right to be angry that they will not get whatever it is over which they are throwing the tantrum?

My granddaughter Lucy just called me. I was asleep in bed. Her ride to high school didn't materialize, and she would be late to school if she walked the one-mile distance. Backstory: Lucy is a great athlete. She does not need more exercise. She's calling me more and more to take her to school, and I often respond because I like to spend the time with her. Yesterday she again called me for a ride home from school, and I was happy to respond, but I had the worry she was developing a coping mechanism of getting others (me) to put out energy rather than expend her own. I started to tell her this, but I couldn't think of a way to say it without impugning her. So, I waited, and this morning I simply responded that I was still asleep. I told her something about me, not her. She walked to school and got there late. I'm trusting that experience to encourage her to not rely on my efforts more than would any lecture. And I got to comfort her that she was late to school instead of scolding her for being "lazy."

A few years ago, Lucy and her sister Darla had no school on a day when their mother was to be at work all day, twenty miles away. They were certainly old enough to spend the day on their own, but it was arranged that I would be "on call" if they had a problem that required adult assistance. I was very angry when I got a call about ten a.m. from Lucy that Darla had thrown a rock and broken a window in her house. I left my house, one half mile away, and walked over after having advised both girls to simply stay away from all broken glass. On the walk, I started out with the idea that I was going to give Darla hell.

As I walked I started to plan the excoriation. Then I hit upon, "What would I tell a patient in this situation?" I would tell the patient that Darla had just learned something she didn't know a moment before. That is not something wrong with her. I realized she would be feeling pretty badly about the whole thing. By the time I got to her house, I was ready to comfort rather than scold her. It turned out she had tossed a pebble to get her sister's attention and everyone was shocked when it left a pockmark in the glass. Nothing had been shattered.

I was amazed that the aspect of the event that disturbed both girls the most was they knew their mother was having a trying day at work, and they were horrified they would add to her distress. They came up with the idea of comforting their mother by doing an especially good job of cleaning the house and having a cold drink and snack ready for her when she came home. They also felt she should learn about the window deficit—which would require replacing a sliding glass door—after she had a chance to decompress from the day's stress. So, they put colorful stickers on the door, one covering the divot and the cracks that were now radiating across the glass. I also comforted Darla with the news that we'd figure out a way that she could earn the money to pay for the door. She was never told she had done anything wrong. She felt closer to me and to her mother for having gone through this event. She will never again throw a rock at a window—unless she intends to break it; I am more sure of that than I would be if she had been scolded, punished, or otherwise abased.

We give children packages of adulthood; hopefully we do this appropriately. Since we will never be totally grown up, it's not possible for us to do so all of the time. But we must try anyway.

One rainy winter day when she was in early primary school, my daughter, Kelly, started out the door to catch the school bus wearing flip flop sandals on her feet. I said to her, "Kelly, it's cold and wet outside. Put on your shoes." She responded, "I want to splash in the puddles," and she ran off for the bus. Now, I could have played the card that I must teach my children obedience, but I think that is sometimes bullying. I decided this was the day to hand Kelly a particular "package" of adulthood. I said nothing. At noon, I got a phone call from Kelly at school. She was crying and said her feet were cold and she wanted me to bring her shoes. I explained I couldn't leave the office, was sad she was uncomfortable, loved her, and I'd see her after school. That evening she told me she had been wrong to have gone to school without proper shoes. I disagreed. She wanted to play in the puddles more than she wanted to have warm feet. I think the problem was not that she was wrong. The problem was her feet got colder than she thought they would. I repeated my attempt to comfort, not scold. She never went off to school again without taking better concern for her comfort. I had decided at that age Kelly could be an adult in regards to her personal comfort in that situation.

When I've told this story, I've been met with criticism for allowing my daughter to suffer. Remember, we live in Southern California and winters are not cold, cool at worst. I would not have handed that package of adulthood to Kelly had we lived in a colder climate. When one hands a package of adulthood to a child, one takes everything into consideration. What works for one kid doesn't work for another. Those decisions are never the same for anyone else. That's why it takes the best judgment one has. I'm only making a plea we don't behave as if the kid is bad or wrong or guilty. It is a perfect kid and the parent must make the judgment call as to when the child is ready for any given piece of adulthood.

How is it a parent has such knowledge as to presume when the child is adult enough for what? Sorry to tell you, that is what parenting is all about. One cannot escape that responsibility. You call it the wisest you see it. But you're there to guide and protect, not to punish and scold.

David Jr. got a package of adulthood forwarded to him at age eighteen, which is absurd because after the eighteenth celebration of one's birth one has all the packages anyway, but it was really cool he knew this and that I was able to recognize it. This little story is one I treasure.

At the time, David was living with me, attending college, and working a job for his own spending money. I was paying his school costs. He had a car, a Suzuki Samurai. He came to me one Thursday telling me he was going to San Francisco for the weekend and wanted to know if I had any advice on activities or sites because I knew the city well. My first response was to tell him he was welcome to take my Chevrolet Blazer for the trip. He'd be more comfortable and safe, and I'd rather not see him take the thousand-mile journey in his tiny car.

He went, had a great trip, and returned. The next weekend he asked if he could borrow my car again because he was again going to San Francisco. I hit the ceiling and told him he was not going to borrow the Blazer because I forbade him to go to San Francisco two weekends in a row. He had school, a job, and limited funds; this second trip was out of the question. David responded exactly the way I hoped he would. There was no conflict whatsoever. He went out, got into his Samurai, and drove to San Francisco. He knew he had that last package of adulthood. It was his car, his school, his money. There was no reason to argue or to have any degree of unhappiness.

So, why did I forbid him to go? I wanted him to go with the knowledge his father thought it a really dumb idea. I also wanted it to be a given that he could disobey authority. He got it. He came back with no sense of rebellion having arisen but with a respect for his time and money that precluded any other trips for a most appropriate period. It was already inherent in our relationship I was not going to disrespect his right to decide for himself and was not going to threaten the "cut off your support" crap. He well knew that my forbidding was no more than a theatric display of my opinion on the matter.

A parent who threatens their adult progeny with, "If you live in my house, you live by my rules," needs to grow up!

One of my favorite possessions is a letter I received from David the following year. He was attending summer school at the University of London and had arrived in England on one of those flights arranged for students at phenomenally cheap prices with the student agreeing to accept destinations near the city and date desired. His flight was booked into Manchester, not London, but he'd arrive in the morning and have time to take a train to his destination before nightfall. The circumstance of the letter was that the airplane arrived twelve hours late, and he was dumped in a strange city, late at night, with no British money and no plans for further transport or lodging.

He started his letter telling me he was angry at me because he did not know what to do, and he thought if I had raised him right he'd know what to do. He said what he had done, though, was ask himself, "What would Dad do if Dad didn't know what to do?" He found a tourist aid desk and asked the woman there, "What would you do if you had just arrived from Los Angeles and didn't know what to do?" That line of reasoning led to his finding help, money, and a B and B in plenty of time to be out dancing in one of Manchester's world-class clubs before midnight. His last sentence was, "So, I guess, Dad, you did raise me right after all."

I've said one hands one's child these little packages of adulthood all through their lives, and by law, the child is totally grown up at eighteen. Clearly I more strongly make the point that one never grows up totally until one is dead. But, under current law, at eighteen the kid can just say, "I'm outta here," and do as they please if they are willing to live with the consequences of doing so. Any parenting one is able to do after the child is eighteen is only with the permission of the kid. In that sense, the child has the ultimate control over himself.

Now, the question behind a tremendous percentage of parent-child conflicts that come to a psychiatrist is how soon does one hand over these packets of adulthood. I believe it is better to hand them over as early as is safe, not as late as is possible.

My older son, John, wanted to go with me one day. He was probably in the seventh grade at the time. I told him I was leaving at five p.m. (several hours off) and I'd take him along if he had a certain chore done. At five he had not started the chore, so I went to leave without him. He said, "If you leave this house without me, I'll burn it down." I said, "Don't, because if you do we'll have no place to live." I left quite wary, but with the certainty I'd rather have my house burned down that day than to have in a few years an adolescent who knew how to blackmail me, so he got a package of adulthood that day. He got to decide whether or not to burn down the house.

I had a friend about that time, who wasn't yet willing to give to her son the "package" of how to behave, how to dress, or how to spend any of his own time—even when to take a crap. That son didn't know how to rebel under such control, except he developed a health-threatening psychosomatic illness that was clearly the only thing about his life his mother could not control. Somehow it happened he just refused to defecate. She took him from doctor to doctor and was totally controlled by her son's resultant megacolon, but even her shrink couldn't get her to ease up on her control of the kid.

I'm happy with how John turned out. I lost track of what happened to the kid who was full of shit. But that's not the point. I respect that the kid is going to turn out according to what the kid is. The parents don't get the credit, positive or negative, for other than what said parents do; the credit for how the kid turns out goes to the kid. However they made out, the parents did the best that they could do with what they—the parents—were.

I clearly wasn't able to follow my own advice during much of my child-rearing years, and that causes me sadness, not guilt. I've told you only a very few stories, and I could tell hundreds of others that would show me to have been no better a parent than most. That's not the point. I'm trying to share ideas to make for child/parent happiness. Sharing stories where I was ignorant and unhappy won't help with that.

To make it easier, let's look back at how it would be if we didn't buy the BS or the SOB and lived as if we were BA and then just did what came naturally. The kid is never wrong. I am never wrong to do what I know to do at that instant. In the next instant I can always do it the way I see to do it in the next instant. I never need to be right. There is no right. I don't blame or accept blame. The kid is welcome to think of me what they want. I'm there to comfort them because I love them and want them to be comforted when they get into trouble. If they get in trouble at school, I comfort them that they are in trouble. I don't debase them because they got into trouble at school. It's not my job to make the problem worse. I also don't interfere or spare them what they got themselves into. I don't bail them out of the consequences, and I support them as they learn from those consequences. Unless...

Unless: If I were to be accused of something of which I were innocent and were facing a court of law, I would hire an attorney. If I were guilty of something but were charged with something more severe than was the fact, I'd hire an attorney. If I were debating the IRS over a dispute that could go either way, I'd hire an attorney. If my dog dug under my neighbor's fence and the neighbor were suing me for ruining their life, I'd hire an attorney. Point made? Were a child of mine to experience a consequence for which I'd normally just comfort him but it now appeared that he needed a parent to step in as an attorney would for a client, then I would go to bat for the kid. You bet I would! But that would be as unusual a situation as it would be for me to hire an attorney.

When I was starting out in practice, I treated Mildred, an anxious, young, single mother of four who was coping marvelously with a very difficult situation, which included her mother telling her that she was doing everything wrong. She saw me for some months and saw that I never blamed her and never blamed her children—or her mother. One day, in a therapy session, she mentioned she had seen me in the grocery, but I had been unaware of her presence. I expressed the wish for her to have felt free to have greeted me and was surprised by her answer that she had not wanted to embarrass me. When I asked her why she thought it would have embarrassed me for her to have said hello, she replied, "Because you were screaming at your children." Enough said about any myth that I can parent better than anybody else.

I treated Oliver, age twelve, when he had disabling anxiety symptoms affecting his physical health. He was the perfect son and was rewarded for being the perfect son, but his anxiety was a clear revelation that he lived in the greatest fear of any imperfection. He reminded me so very much of me at that age. I worked with Oliver's parents to try to get them to drop the insistence of everything having to be perfect. I held my composure, but almost shrieked, when one day they told me of a battle they'd had with him when he was just beginning to loosen up and wanted to spend his own allowance money on a bicycle part they felt was of poor quality. They had stopped him from buying it, and on another occasion, they had forbade him to skip a chorus practice in an extracurricular activity at which he'd accrued a perfect attendance and on-time record. He was clearly suffering, but they could only complain that these examples showed how he needed their continued control. I knew the situation was fragile, but I was still disappointed and saddened when I was unsuccessful to get them to back off one iota, and they pulled him out of therapy. I learned from that experience of the need to be a more gentle therapist than I had been with them. Maybe I was being too direct with them, as direct as I wished someone had been with my parents.

Everything I have said about the child is also true about the parent. Everything one has done as a parent–as a person–was the best that one knew to do at that moment. To have done any better, a parent would have had to have been wiser, more knowledgeable, more patient, more rich in resources than was possible for that parent to have been at any given instant.

A forty-seven-year-old woman came to see me because she didn't know how to deal with a crisis. She came in wringing her hands and crying. Her son's girlfriend was pregnant, and they were planning to marry when clearly (to anyone except them) marriage would be creating a huge problem rather than solving one–they were not marriage material. They had been making love when it would have been better to have been sport fucking and now were trapped in the beginnings of misery. Timing is everything. I listened an appropriate amount of time (how I ever got that right, I'll never know) before saying, "Wow, well, I'll bet you're glad that isn't your problem." She looked like I had shot her; then she laughed, saw the point, and we began therapy. Herein lies a big issue for parents. She didn't know she could love and comfort her son while he was caught in his problem. She just assumed it was her problem. Poor boy hadn't gotten enough packets of adulthood along the way. I endorsed her doing anything that she knew to do to help the kid but to keep it in the category of problems he was having, not that she was having. It is a joy to be able to do whatever it is we can to help an adult offspring who is in over their head. It is sad to become anxious when we think it is our failure if we can't fix their problems.

A pediatrician was addressing a parent forum when a woman asked the doctor at what age she should start educating her child about sex. The speaker was, I think, using my technique of being dramatic to make the point when he asked the woman when this child would be born. The woman, taken aback, answered that the child was five years old, to which the pediatrician retorted, "Good God, woman, what are you doing sitting here? Get home and get started. You are five years late already."

Too many Americans are as puritanical as the Puritans who were too crazy for Europe and got ejected in the seventeenth Century. On this side of the pond they lacked natural enemies, so they thrived and still influence what we do to our children. There is a big difference between being natural about bodies and sex and being abusive, and Americans aren't very good about finding that gap.

A few years ago the San Clemente police were called to the beach, and child services got involved when a prude saw a naked baby on a beach towel being kissed on the buttocks by their parents. A valley woman was shown on the evening news saying, "What if my children were to see that?" when speaking in protest to a mosaic being installed at LAX that included male nudity—a mosaic for god's sake! Art museum docents pay attention to easing school children into exhibits that include nude figures. There are still books in print that tell boys they are harming themselves to masturbate. What crap! It's no wonder that adolescent sexual behavior causes more mischief in America than it does in civilized countries.

Limits can be set on behaviors that do not require children to be taught that they are nasty. Looking into another child's pants may be normal exploration, not perversion, even though it may have more of a sexual basis than adults realize exists in young children. Grade school boys are not going to be ruined if they are not beaten for espying a *Hustler* magazine.

I treated a woman in her fifties who was amazingly fragile emotionally. Her son was a patient of mine, and he got her to come see me. The pain that mother had suffered since early childhood was palpable. I'm not so simple as to think the following was the cause of her psychiatric diagnoses, but it took her weeks of being schooled in freeing herself from blame/shame before she told me that the central abhorrence that had been choking her soul for four dozen years had been her involvement in a pre-puberty sex game, which was entirely non-pathological and should have been a fun memory of childhood. Her demeanor changed, and she made good progress in therapy with that shame out of the way.

We really screw up our kids when we are afraid to let them hate us. David Jr. once told me he was furious with me because I had not been enough of a bastard for him to be angry with me like his friends were angry with their fathers. He thought he'd missed out on an important experience. Geez! You can't win! Kelly needed some encouragement when she rued that her kids sometimes hated her. She has now come to see that was all natural. Her daughters have developed fabulously and she has wonderful relationships with both of them. Adolescence is so fluid that some days your kids are in Group A and other days in Group B.

I use a metaphor that children are like water. You cannot push or pull them, but if you build dams and survive the force when they crash into you, you can direct their flow.

I diagnosed many twenty-year-old "children" as having Mission Viejo Syndrome. A common demographic of the city where I practiced consisted of parents who had far more money than that with which they were raised. To see themselves as good, they had to provide for their kids all they had wished for in their own adolescences. I could well have supported myself on just treating young adults who were given everything by parents who then saw it as their duty to make them shape up by scolding and demeaning. The kids would come to see me following high school, having dropped out of college, without jobs, and getting into all of the troubles brought on by having no judgment about behavior or consequences, and they'd come to see me in their new 'Vettes, BMWs, and Shelby Mustangs. Parents saw it as their job to control and motivate—to guilt and to shame—their kids but could only have pride in themselves if they gave their children everything.

The ultimate was the college dropout whose parents could not get him off the couch, couldn't even get him to turn off the lights or lock the door before he went to bed or to put his dishes in the sink. He came in late for his fourth session because his parents had taken away his Corvette the day before. They had replaced it with a Porsche, which the kid didn't know how to shift.

39

What Do the Simple Folk Do?

"JUDGE NOT, that ye be..." has a meaning for me that really has nothing to do with hypocrisy or sin. It has to do with being happy. To the extent I am able to escape the BS (I am wrong to not be better than I am) for myself and on behalf of every other human, the world becomes so very much a happier place for me.

I often tried to make sense of the quotation, "I never met a man I didn't like." In my childhood, I'd search to name some human whom Will Rogers would have not liked. I came up with Dillinger, Stalin, Leopold and Loeb, or the guy who killed Charles Lindbergh Jr. I do suppose Rogers never met any of those people, but he certainly would have known of them all. Now I see, Rogers could only have been talking about himself. He had the belief he could find something likable in anyone. Or maybe I'm all wrong. Maybe he hated lots of people but just never met them, or maybe he lied.

I love the story of the woman who said she could say something nice about anybody. She was challenged to apply that to the devil. She thought for a moment, then with a grin said, "Well, at least he's persistent."

Obviously a lot of people have traits I don't like. I have some very good friends whom I don't like. Some of them bore me, some offend my nose, and with some I'm embarrassed to be seen. We're friends because we have a long history together; I can always count on them, and I'm willing to always be there for them. I just don't want to spend much time with them. But another reason I maintain the friendship is I see my dissatisfaction with them to be a statement about me, not about them. If I'm afraid to be seen with them, it's because I'm socially insecure. If they bore me, it's because I'm so boring I need to be entertained. The nose, well, maybe it speaks for me not...No, they just stink, but that's really a minor problem in the overall of life.

Before getting the gist of the BA process, I'd see anyone who abused substances as a bad person. Now, I understand I needed to see myself as good for not using drugs, and how could I do that unless I saw as bad anyone who did? Anyone different from me in any way had to be seen as bad if I wanted to see myself as good. Since endorsing being BA, I realize everyone is doing the best they can with what they've got, and I shan't fault myself nor them no matter what the other's predilections. When I am able to think about it—which is not all the time—I remember to stop facilitating the SOB and realize I don't need to make them wrong to make me right.

Sheila was a friend for many years. I admired her intelligence, her ability to make good places for herself in life, and her many friends whom she was always happy to share. Then one day Sheila asked me to do something which would have been a violation of my medical ethics. I explained that was something I was not willing to do, and she threw a hissy fit. I should do it because of our friendship. We were at a party when this disruption in our harmony occurred, and she didn't speak or make eye contact with me the rest of the evening. We had plans two days hence to run a mutual errand. I called her and told her I'd be by to pick her up at ten thirty. We behaved together that day as if the previous event had not occurred. To me, it wasn't worth anything because I simply saw it as if she had a brain fart. I've had lots of those and saw no reason to let it interfere in our friendship. I had not argued with her and had not labeled her ethics. I simply had told her I was not willing to do what she had wanted me to do. The conflict evaporated. Some weeks later, she initiated, "I don't know what happened on that night." I countered I didn't either. That was the end of it. Our friendship had survived an all-out assault because I had not felt assaulted. I had simply witnessed my friend having an eruption, though it had been a surprise to me. However, I never again had the level of trust in our relationship I had before because I knew that she would have been willing to destroy the friendship rather than admit that she was wrong (a concept I wouldn't have acknowledged anyway).

Years later we got to talking about past relationships, Sheila and I, to an extent we had not previously ventured. She told me story after story of deep, long-lasting, intimate, loving relationships she had abandoned because she couldn't get the other person to see they were wrong—and she was right—about something. When I saw this about Sheila, I realized I was putting more time and attention into our relationship than I cared to. We saw much less of each other, but the relationship remained cordial, so cordial, in fact, that we planned a trip together a few years after the above event. On that trip, Sheila stunned me by asking me how I could not believe in a god when I saw the beauty of the flowers. The beauty of the flowers? OK, I'm not taking on creationism at this point, but come on. Sheila was an educated person with advanced degrees, and she brought up this argument I hadn't heard since grade school. A little later, on that same trip, she started telling me which roads she thought I should take to get to a destination although she knew I was very familiar with the area—to which she had never been before. OK, now the explosion at the party over my medical ethics, the ending of friendships because she couldn't get friends to see they were wrong, along with her inability to see what was and was not infantile about her beliefs really bored me.

I've only seen Sheila once in the last five years. That was on an occasion about four and a half years ago in which she brought to my house some friends with whom she wanted to impress me. I was only impressed that she was trying to impress me, and I've never seen her since. But were I to walk up to her, I would see our friendship as intact. I wish her no harm. I'd do what I could to make her comfortable or help her out. I just find she is no one with whom I want to spend time. I have friends whom I enjoy immensely. I spend all the time I can with them because of the fun I get from being with them. I don't rank any of them above or below Sheila as persons.

Another example of how understanding the principles of part 2 make me a happier person occurred the night before I wrote this chapter. A good friend accused me of something which was preposterous. I dug down and resisted my surface impulse to defend myself, going instead for what I preach and therefore ought to believe and practice. I was then really grateful because he showed me my behavior had been vague and could be interpreted by intelligent people to mean exactly what I had no intention of meaning. I feel closer to him than before his accusation. And I feel no urge to argue the point. It's OK for him to see it as best he knows how to see it. By my valuing his opinion, I suspect that he feels closer to me than before it was I did or didn't do what he thought I did. Of course, I'd take a different action were I being accused of a crime or some other matter of significance. But wouldn't it be great (happier) if I were able to feel the way I do now, even if I were preparing a legal defense?

I recently found this quotation: "I never knew how strong I was until I had to forgive someone who wasn't sorry and accept an apology I never received." I doubt that Anonymous is a happy person. Anonymous sounds more self-righteous than happy. I've never had to forgive anyone and no one has ever owed me an apology.

Some people have shown themselves to be in Group A, others in Group B, and by far, most people oscillate between groups. Some people have made me sad; some have made me angry. But when I can remember what is in part 2, I can just decide what part of my life I want to share with them. It's as simple as that. True apologies and forgiveness don't belong in a happy life. Caring, acceptance, and expressions of sadness do.

No person is good or bad enough to be my friend or to be axed off my friend list. I simply do what I'm willing to do with all the opportunities I have with other travelers through a mostly joyful life.

"Never complain; Never explain."

BENJAMIN DISRAELI

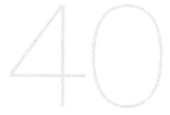

9 to 5

I REALLY DID ENJOY MY TIME in the Navy. I detested the war, found the Marines to be rigid, and hated having been drafted. But I was happy. I liked treating the patients, found the legal and administrative work to be interesting, felt competent, and thrived with the stimulation of the challenges. I sparred with several of the colonels over marines whom they wanted to punish and I wanted to treat. I always won. After all, I was the Navy psychiatrist. There was one of me; there were multitudes of them. I technically had the power to sign a paper and have any of them carted off to the Navy Hospital Psychiatric Unit. But the thing most significant and important to me was getting to live with my family, in my home, while my draft obligation was fulfilled.

In the clinic where I worked there were four other physicians doing general medical work. They were miserable and ever complaining. I was feeling sorry for them until I realized the very things about which they groused applied equally to me. Then I really felt sorry for them. They did not have the ability to enjoy what I enjoyed, even though those things applied equally to them. To be fair, they were younger than I and had been physicians for less years than I had, and I'm sure that made a difference. They were needing to prove something about themselves not about to be recognized by the Navy. They felt their required compliance with Navy procedure treaded on their autonomy; their attention was focused on this and other slights built into the system. All of this applied equally to me, but my attention was focused on the fact I got to be with my family and serve out my draft obligation at the same time. This was also true for them. Their focus was on their prestige; mine was on how pleasant and easy was my life. We were all in the same situation, but what we experienced was divergent. It was *Rashomon*.

They were irate their expertise couldn't counter Navy policy. I would have been happy to have straightened paper clips for two years to get out of the military unscathed. Needless to say, the Navy command was very happy with me and very unhappy with them, but that was quite irrelevant to us docs.

One of my favorite stories from my years in private practice centers on Ruth, who hated her boss with a passion. She wouldn't leave the job because she could not find another that would pay as well. Without her level of pay she couldn't afford her house, and she'd rather live with the obnoxious boss than leave her home. So, anger management for Ruth was to concentrate on how angry she was at her boss for several moments and then to concentrate on all the things she loved about where she lived. She, in short time, became a happy person who hated her boss and loved her house. She was at peace with her anger. She didn't need to change anything. She didn't need to get even. It became, for the sake of her house, OK with her to live the rest of her career being angry at her boss and loving her house.

One might ask if it's healthy to work for years for a boss at whom one is angry. I'd say yes if one is OK with being angry–sees it as a normal part of life and not a sign they are a victim if they can't "fix" it. They have to reject the BS about anger and stay away from the SOB. And, of course, when it just becomes not worth it for the house, then one quits the job, sues for discrimination, shoots the boss–whatever one, with good judgment, is willing to live with the consequences of doing. Ruth was happy with her progress; she terminated therapy and within a short time had moved away–from the boss and the house.

A few years on a man came to see me who had never had any contact with or knowledge of Ruth but who, by coincidence, was now working for Ruth's old boss. He was depressed. He felt he would be less depressed if he could get away from that boss. One day, as an aside, he told me many employees in the company had signs on their desks that read, "I love my house." I had treated the whole damn company for years to come when Ruth had been my patient!

There's an important lesson here about responsibility. If you are doing something, you do want to do it. Maybe a gun is pointed at you; maybe your house is at stake; maybe you are alone and pregnant; maybe she has got you by the balls. If you hate the situation, really hate it, get really, really angry at it but understand you get to do what you want to about it. You will be a mentally healthier person than if you feel trapped. This belief is bolstered by memoirs written in later years by survivors of Nazi labor and death camps.

Sometimes power comes from admitting you are unable to make a decision. I was in a situation once in which I was helped by something a patient taught me after I had shown it to her, but I didn't see it for myself until she got it and fed it back to me.

Julie had been in a great deal of emotional pain when her job provided her with desired benefits and a career path that thrilled her; she was treated very well and liked her boss, but she questioned the ethical foundation of the business. Questioned was the right word. She wasn't sure there was a problem over which she'd want to leave the company, but her suspicion there might be became the perceived basis for much anxiety. One day she announced she was undecided about the job and decided to not act until she was decided. Her anxiety dropped significantly, and soon she decided to leave.

About the time she left, I encountered a life crisis that was eased when I said to myself that I was undecided, and my decision was to do nothing as long as I was undecided. When I decided, then I'd do something. There was actually some degree of peace of mind by reaffirming that the control was mine, even in my indecision.

41

My Favorite Things

IT IS CLEAR ONE CAN NEVER HAVE ENOUGH to make one happy if happiness is based on having enough. Richard Nixon held the most powerful position in the world, but it was his need for more power that led to his crimes and his disgrace. Marilyn Monroe is said to have been haunted by the belief she was not beautiful enough. You might have enough money with which to be happy, but there are billionaires who need more.

The symbols are ever changing across society, and each person has their own. There are men of any degree of financial wealth who need more wealth simply to compensate because their cock isn't larger. In Anthony Weiner's case it is more than big enough, but appropriate behavior was impossible as long as there were still people who hadn't seen it. There are women of great beauty who must have one more plastic surgery, and they've been made to look ridiculous. There are people of average appearance and means whose happiness depends on one more academic accolade. Geez, look at the athletes with to-die-for bodies who have steroided themselves into infamy or death because they couldn't accept the level at which they performed. Or, do tell, how ridiculous do notable scientists look to the less famous when they squabble about the publicity they do or don't get for their discoveries?

Octomom wasn't content with six children. Richard Angelo's fragile ego couldn't settle for being a competent nurse; he killed twenty-five patients so he could bring them back with heroics at Good Samaritan (!) Hospital in New York.

I do hate to be a bore, but the need to be Born Again comes into view once again. Rather than going through life believing there is good and bad and that somehow we need to be better than we are–line up the popsicle sticks: good = strong = powerful = big cock = D cup bra = tight pussy = money = beautiful = smart = famous = holy = pious = educated, etc.–the way to escape into true happiness is to start over with the understanding no one is any better or any worse than anyone else, and the adoration of symbols is just a compensation for neuroses. If you are a happy person, you spend your life enjoying every moment and doing the things that are available to you to do because of the joy those things bring you. What you don't get, you don't get to enjoy. What you do get, you do get to enjoy. But you don't change what you think of you, whether you enjoy getting it or don't enjoy not getting it.

I enjoy the taste of a really good apple. I hate the taste of a really bad apple. I love a roller coaster ride. I hate a train wreck. But the joy or horror of the experience does not need to change my sense of myself. My ego can be the same whether I am grieving, furious, pleased, or elated about an external happening if I am a truly happy, healthy individual–admittedly an ideal which has never been 100 percent reached by anyone.

When I was in medical school I spent about the same amount of money on a car as did my friends who bought ordinary, modest new cars. However, the car I bought was a lovely, old, highly depreciated Rolls-Royce–a tiny model that once had been made in very small numbers and had earlier belonged to Mary Pickford. I never could afford to restore it to the point of making it a treasure. It was too old, too tiny, and too deteriorated to be any kind of a status symbol–that was the thing I liked about it–but it was a lot of fun and was the source of stories which are still fun to tell. Years later I quite actually had to choose between the wife and the car, and I made the wrong choice. About three years after selling the car and buying what my then growing family could afford, I ran into a friend whom I had not seen in five years.

He said, "David, do you still drive the Rolls-Royce?" I answered, "No, I sold it and bought a Volkswagen." He said, "I didn't know a person could do that." My reply was, "I liked my car better when I had the Rolls-Royce, but I like myself the same in either car."

A humorous anecdote happened a couple of decades later. A friend from the old days who had sucked up to me because I had a Rolls-Royce ran into me shortly after he had bought a new Ferrari. He feigned great interest in me in asking what I was driving, and I knew it would be his glorification to top whatever I might answer with the news of his Italian masterwork. He was absolutely crestfallen when I answered I was driving an old Buick. He could tell I would not care a used tinker's dam about being one-upped. One cannot use a new Ferrari to trump another who is happy in an old Buick.

I have never made a study of Eastern religions. I should. I should have before starting this book. I didn't. I've heard enough about some of them to believe what I'm about to say is what some of them, in part, teach. I believe the practitioners of same would not read this book because they already know what it is that I'm trying to say. But I'm writing for the rest of us. I do not believe in the twenty-first century in the western world these concepts need to be embedded in a philosophy or religion.

Happiness has nothing to do with how much in life is desirable or undesirable. I maintain the less we notice ourselves, the happier we will become. If I am poor, the lack of wealth is a smaller impediment to happiness than is the sense that I am nothing, have failed, am less than another, deserve what I don't have, or blame myself for my choices. The other end of that sick popsicle stick is just as disturbing—that I am something, have succeeded, am more than another, or deserve what I have if I am rich.

I have a friend who lost the ends of two fingers in an accident. A year later he told me he wasn't bothered by the missing digital pieces, but he was very bothered by—and couldn't shake—the sense there was something wrong with him, that he was defective. My friend from some pages above, the one who is happy that he can count to twenty-one on his body, is always focused on doing something that he enjoys. His sense that he can do something overrides any sense of what he is. What he is is a given. I can't draw conclusions over which one of them is happier, but I do believe that "I am damaged" is a "to be" thought that is disturbing. "I will act" is a "to do" thought which can bring pleasure.

If climbing a mountain is all about me being a mountain climber, I aver the joy is not as complete as it would be if it were all about the exercise, the view, the mountain, etc. If I don't make it to the top, I'm a happier person if I grieve I didn't see the view from the top—or I didn't get the scout ribbon or I broke my leg—than if I have just become a mountaineering failure.

I teach happiness or misery has a lot to do with what one pays attention to. This may be learned or inborn—let's leave that to the philosophers and researchers—but, whichever, it can be nurtured to some extent. I can learn, at least in part, to concentrate on the beauty of the new car more and on that dent less. Of course, to do this I have to not be blaming myself for the dent or feeling helpless I can't punish the crone who opened her car door into mine. (Yeah, if I could smash her car I'd feel better.) Let's get back to the idea it isn't about whether or not I was good enough, bold enough, careful enough, vengeful enough. Let's just get back to enjoying all the things I love about the car and hating the dent. That is a happier state.

If my life is 85 percent the way I want it and I concentrate on the other 15 percent I will be unhappy. If my life is 85 percent the way I don't want it, I will be happy if I concentrate on the 15 percent that is the way I want it. This principle is true whatever are the numbers in the ratio.

There are persons in prisons, on deathbeds, or in miserable marriages whom we could still see as being happy. We read in the celebrity press of those who have everything, every thing that could be desired—including accolades and fame—and are clearly unhappy people.

If I am jealous of what you have, I'm not unhappy because I don't have what you have. I'm unhappy because I am jealous.

I am sure that if I can have the attitudes expressed in this chapter, I will be happier with my looks than was Monroe, with my power than was Nixon, and with my wealth than was Midas. I have enough sex appeal, consequence, and money to be happy; they didn't.

Catherine was a wealthy businesswoman; she was as flamboyant as she was successful—new money all the way; she had made it herself. I was seeing her because she suffered more anxiety than she was willing to abide. One day the subject of her session was her angst since her CPA told her she would have to sell either her Rolls-Royce or her Ferrari. (I never subjected her to hearing my R-R story.) It was clear that either car was not the issue. The issue was that she would no longer be Catherine the Great, the woman who conquered a male-dominated career so completely that she could drive both the world's best sedan and the world's best sports car! (This story happened years before Maybach and Bugatti reappeared on the scene.)

My dad was in the doctor's parking lot at Palm Harbor Hospital in Garden Grove on the morning in late September 1960 when the Ford Motor Company was to unveil its new and totally over-the-top Lincoln Continental—the complete departure from all previous luxury cars that soon became known as the Kennedy Lincoln when our thirty-fifth president rode frequently and died in one. Somehow, Dr. Leggett, the reigning orthopedic surgeon in the region, had managed to arrive at work in one hours before the showroom would open. When Henry Louria, a respected and better grounded general surgeon, pulled up in his aging Hillman Minx, the contrast in values was palpable and painful to hoi polloi gathered around the Lincoln. In a futile attempt to lessen the tension, Leggett called out, "Where's your status symbol, Hank?" To which Louria replied, "Right behind my zipper where it belongs."

"The mind is its own place,
and in itself
Can make a Heav'n of Hell,
a Hell of Heav'n."

John Milton

42

Get Me to the Church On Time

MY TWO P.M. PATIENT RUSHED IN, OUT of breath, at 2:02 and began sputtering out an apology and excuses for why she was late. She was clearly upset and—germane to this book—was unhappy with herself. We'll call her Joan.

DS: "Why are you apologizing?"

Joan: "Because I'm late."

DS: "You're not late. Why are you apologizing?"

Joan: "I should have been here before two."

DS: "Sez who?"

Joan: "That was the time I was supposed to be here."

DS: "Joan, you booked an appointment with me from two until two fifty. I'm going to charge you for that time, but that doesn't obligate you to anything. I don't want to see you be taken advantage of, but you surely don't owe it to me to come at any particular time."

Joan: "You're weird! My last psychiatrist would scold me if I were late."

DS: "That has nothing to do with you. You've just described two doctors, and I happen to think it was he who was weird, not I."

Joan was in therapy for a few months and made great progress in becoming a happier, less anxious person. About four months after that two p.m. visit, she waltzed in seven minutes "late," her second time at not being there ten minutes before the hour. She was acknowledging her progress by sharing with me without apology, "I was having lunch with a friend, and I decided I wanted a second cup of coffee and a forty-three-minute session more than I wanted a fifty-minute session and one cup of coffee."

I grew up in a family that was always late. My mother set the agendas, and she was always late, so the whole family was late. After I left home, I did a lot better than she on this score and was only late about 85 percent of the time. I was ever rushing, always trying to get something done, often cutting corners and always apologizing because I knew it was "bad" to be late. To the extent I was able to manage the BA experience, this began to change. It did not change because I became more aware or guilt ridden about being late. It changed because I began to practice what I was learning from my patients. I'll acknowledge Joan as having helped me in this matter.

One day a companion was prodding me to go faster and I blurted out, "I don't have time to hurry!" I had never been aware of that thought, not even an instant before I said it. My friend laughed and it became a motto for me to hang on to. Interestingly, my being late decreased by more than 50 percent. Most of the time I had been late, it was because I was hurrying to get something done. When the motto sank in, it prevented me from starting anything unless I had ample time to see it finished. Now I am calmer, more relaxed and in that state get more done and am late less often. I metaphorically give myself the option of the second cup of coffee and the forty-three-minute session whenever I want, but like Joan that happens a small minority of the time.

One day in the office, I asked my secretary to do something and returned a few moments later to find she had done what I had asked of her. I was stunned. She didn't understand my being surprised; she was an efficient woman who expected me to expect it would be done. What that experience showed me was that I was going through life putting "on the list" anything I needed done. I had expected her to put what I had asked on the list of things to do. She had, instead, just done it. What stunned me was my sudden enlightenment as to why I was always disorganized and late.

Believing being late and not getting things done to be bad while trying hard to be good was useless. Giving myself the option to do as I wanted to do based only on what consequences I wanted to live with has helped.

The BS teaches us to be proud of ourselves when we don't put off until tomorrow anything we can do today and to do well anything worth doing. Ripping away the BS and being willing to not obey, to not get pride involved, and to understand that blame is an SOB frees one to put off until tomorrow anything that doesn't have to be done today and to accept that a lot of things are worth doing half-assed. A more important corollary is that no task should be given your all. Don't put more effort into anything than it is worth to you. Otherwise, you'll be putting your life into things that actually have a limited value.

I also learned in college that procrastinating is not such a bad thing. There were assignments on which I'd start to work a week before they were due. I found that those assignments then took one full week. If I started the assignment four hours before it was due, it took four hours. Then I came to understand that any task expands to fill whatever time is available for it.

Another significant, time-related issue resolved by being Born Again is that of waiting in lines or sitting in traffic. The reason for the intense irritation of seeing the other line move faster involves two things: 1) actual, usually insignificant, grief that one is delayed for a few seconds and 2) the blame one puts on oneself for having chosen the wrong lane, which may be defended against by blaming another—the slow person ahead in line. This may seem too trivial for me to have called it significant until one realizes how much unhappiness one sees in slow lines and in traffic. Some just can't stand the unfairness or loss of pride of seeing themselves in the slow lane. This became tragic to my family when a close friend, Loren, was murdered at age twenty-five in a road rage incident wherein neither Loren nor his killer could stand the loss of pride in having his position challenged.

43

Over the Rainbow

I WAS PRETTY MUCH THROUGH with my early childhood when we got our first television. Before that I remember a salesman coming to our house and demonstrating a garbage disposal by grinding up a Coca-Cola bottle and sending its sand into the city sewer. One day my dad brought home a ballpoint pen. We had never seen such a thing. I ran its line all over a page for what seemed like a much longer time than it really was and marveled I couldn't get it to run out of ink. I remember dumping the household trash in a cement thingy at the farthest corner of the backyard and burning it—the trash, not the yard or the thingy. I remember not being able to swim in public pools because of the danger of polio. A school chum of mine helped to tend his physician father who was confined to an iron lung because of that virus. In his life-giving coffin his dad had become certified in the interpretation of EKG squiggles and had been able to support the family modestly by dictating reports while his son or wife held the tracings where he could see them.

As a natural consequence of my father's unwillingness to discard anything and the Schroeder travel gene, a stack of *National Geographic* magazines metastasized through our tiny apartment, later throughout the small house my parents bought in 1947. It is a scientifically proven fact when the world comes to an end it will be as the result of the earth's crust being crushed by the weight of NG magazines. What else? They will be printed forever, and none will ever be thrown away. At least that was the doctrine that my family was supporting—much more romantic and less scary than global warming or nuclear winter as the pet panic of that day.

I poured through those magazines for hours, years on end as a child. All the time a kid of today spends on TV + soccer + video games was rolled into my studying every copy in that jungle of issues going all the way back to the mid part of WWI—or the Great War as it then was. Every fact taught years later in my high school geography and history classes was something I had learned before going to kindergarten. Yes, of course, finding pictures of naked natives on far-off islands was also part of the fun—boobs and butts and balls.

A few years ago I realized I have traveled to all of the sites about which I can remember being enthralled in the 1940s except the Taj Mahal. It became important for me to get to Agra before senility set in, until I realized that were I to get there I would succeed at having done as a seventy-year-old man what a seven-year-old kid had set as a goal. What a disgusting idea! A man could, at the end of his life, still be letting a seven-year-old child who had lived during the Truman administration ru(i)n his life! I feel as if I've grown more in traveling the world to see all kinds of places I'd never even considered before I actually went there. Next year, I want to be led by the man I am next year, not the boy I was seven decades ago.

Now, I do realize it would be great to see India, and the Taj Mahal must be marvelous. But I had recently been feeling unless I saw it I would have failed—at seeing all those things that boy of sixty-eight years ago had determined to see. The brightest I can be today may not be what I thought was worth being back in that day of inkwells, radio dramas, garbage pails, iron lungs, incinerators, and yellowed, old, yellow magazines.

This principle is ubiquitous. I am responsible for what I do now and cannot cop out that I am successful to have done something I had earlier determined to do. If at 12:03 I decide that I no longer want to do what I had planned for today at 8:51, then I am a happier person to drop it and move on. Maybe I've failed if, at the end of the day, I have finished all I had planned to do at the beginning of the day.

Only do those things that are (present tense) worth doing; don't do anything for the sake of self-improvement or to fulfill a goal. That doesn't mean don't increase your skills and it doesn't mean don't stick to things, even if they are hard and take a long time. Just realize it won't make you better to do something you don't now think is worth doing.

The same thought also helped me to stop being as much of a hoarder as I had been. One day I realized the only reason I was saving some souvenirs was because I had already saved them for fifty years; I tossed them. Once, without realizing until later what a charming adage it was for an anal-compulsive, I blurted out to a friend who was explaining why he was saving an old knickknack, "Yes, and if you save your shit for three thousand years, you'll have three-thousand-year-old shit."

My happiness in the future rests on my knowledge that when I am eighty-nine I will look back and see what a fool I was at eighty-eight–happiness because that will mean I am still growing. I do not need to fear that I will be unhappy with me whatever happens regarding the goals of yore, be they met or unmet.

Therapy is like a tennis lesson. You don't tell the student to "hit the ball." You teach them how to hold the racket, then how to begin the swing, then how to maintain the position of the wrist through the swing, etc. You don't tell someone to not "feel badly" about the unsatisfied past dreams. You teach them all the stuff we've covered earlier in this book. Then the way to help becomes clear. It also helps the psychotherapist if they believe what they are saying. There is valid reason to feel grief and sadness at looking at the past. There is no reason to feel guilt or shame or blame or loss of self-esteem at looking at the past.

Patients have taught me a great part of fear of death is that they don't want to die having failed to meet those expectations they have had of themselves. Fear of the future is often a manifestation of that same theme. I remember when I was a young father, I thought if I were to die I would have failed. This was different than wanting my kids to not be orphaned. That thought was about them, but there was the other about me not succeeding in what I wanted to do with them. In the movie, Philomena needed to not die until she had found her son.

As a young man seeing the Acropolis over the left wing of a BEA Comet, which was making a banked turn as it was arriving in Athens, I entertained a very conscious thought that if the plane crashed on landing it would be OK because I had seen the Parthenon. That wasn't a romantic thought. It was infantile and obscene—that for me to die or not to die would be OK or not OK depending on whether or not I had fulfilled a child's distant fantasy.

I would feel self-centered telling you about these neuroses of mine except my patients taught me they had them, too. I'm writing them because I don't think they're just about me; they are about my readers as well. Lucile put the kibosh on my fear of dying before I had grown up when she was undaunted, even happy, with the way she handled that *faux pas* in the restaurant at ninety-two.

With apologies to Ernie Pyle and Dwight Eisenhower, I hasten to proclaim that there most certainly are atheists in foxholes. Let my religion or lack of it be related to what I believe about the unknown; I don't need a cover for a neurotic fear that I'm not good enough and a celestial comeuppance is lying in ambush for me beyond the stars.

I have heard that existential depression occurs in mankind because humans, alone, understand they are going to die. Duh! Humans get depressed over death because humans, alone, have been falsely taught they will die because they weren't good enough. Back to the hair splitting, folks. Anyone may well be sad they will die. They may be angry they will die. But depression only comes from the pollution of their minds with the ideas of failure. I won't repeat it, but go back and consider that anecdote about airplane anxiety in chapter 12.

The BS tells you every misfortune or unmet purpose is because of some inadequacy—on the part of you or (SOB) of someone or something else. The toy broke because you weren't careful enough. My mother told me if I didn't stop farting no girl would want me. Any pain in your career is because you didn't study hard enough, work hard enough, seduce the right person on the way up, pray hard enough, or judge the job market carefully enough. Not enough. Not enough. Every marital problem is because you weren't kind enough, weren't enough of a judge of human nature in choosing your mate, didn't listen to your mother well enough, don't have a big enough bust or penis, didn't make enough of your career. Or else your problem is the fault of Mattel, a parent, a boss, a god, government manipulation of the economy, a conniving rat, or an immigrant.

You are going to die. Period. That's it folks; no reason for depression. Now get out there and enjoy every moment, every decade you've got.

There may be a lot of future between now and demise. We can make sure it is as happy as possible for whatever it is that happens by remembering to be willing to fear but never to worry. Remember to be angry or sad when you don't have what you want but to never let the fear of disappointment keep you from going after everything that you want. Remember that every moment of your life you have done the best you could do, and what comes next is something not deserved but is something that is or is not opportune.

I remember some decades ago reading about a reply that Zelda Fitzgerald had made to a question about her philosophy of life. I have not been able to find reference to it in recent years, so maybe it is coming from me and I'm just giving her the blame or credit for the quote: "I go after everything I want, and what I don't get, I do without." It is as simple as that.

A lot has been said about the wisdom that comes with age. Nonagenarians get it. For the rest of us, we have to keep at it—at the task of getting better and better at learning that we don't need to be better.

"The future ain't what it used to be."

YOGI BERRA

44

Purpose

LET'S TRY TO GET RID OF the manifestations of the BS for a moment. You are not here for any task that obligates you to keep on living until it's done. There is no reason you are here. The cause for you being here is your biological father knocked up your biological mother. Maybe ancillary factors are a condom broke or they wanted a child or someone was drunk. Or maybe someone wanted to get pregnant to manipulate a situation. (Of course, there are other possibilities like in vitro fertilization, artificial insemination, and immaculate conception, but these are not the causes for the existence of the majority of my readers.)

For a hundred thousand years or decades, H. sapiens have been working on civilization and haven't got it right yet. We don't have an economic system that works, an educational system that works, or a government that works, and we don't yet know how to raise children—even worse, get along with each other. And we've never reached any consensus about from where we came or if we are going anywhere.

One of the handful of classic cartoon themes is the scenario of a student climbing to the mountaintop to ask a guru what is the meaning of life. The multiplicity of such cartoons is only a testimony to the ubiquity of our philosophical thirst.

In my thinking, I have eschewed the subjects of how many angels can fit on the head of a pin, determinism versus free will, the existence of the gods, and a number of other subjects I feel only fools rush in to. I do believe the cosmologists who aver the ultimate question remains, "Why is there anything?"

Paul, a physician colleague of mine, told me the following story: he had a patient, Mickey, who was hard drinking, obese, and diabetic; he smoked cigarettes, never exercised, and was married to a manipulator. Mickey died of a heart attack in his late forties. Paul was amazed, but not surprised, when he was served a subpoena to testify in a civil trial in which the Shrew was suing Mickey's most recent employer in a wrongful death suit alleging stress at work. On the stand, Paul was asked by the plaintiff's attorney why Mickey had died. Paul summarized Mick's lack of compliance with any medical advice or common sense and explained how diabetes, obesity, lack of exercise, and smoking combined with genetic factors might lead to a cardiac catastrophe. The attorney, going after some legal principle which I do know about but don't care much about in this case, persisted over and over after each of Paul's replies, "Yes, but why did he die?" Paul didn't know of any job stress that might have contributed, and he wasn't about to bring up the marriage. Finally, he just looked at the attorney and said, "Counselor, we don't know why anything happens. We know that the sun comes up in the morning; we know how the sun comes up in the morning, but we don't know why the sun comes up in the morning. We know that rain falls from the sky; we know how rain falls from the sky, but we don't know why rain falls from the sky. We know that occasionally an idiot gets through law school and passes the bar; we know how the idiot gets through law school and passes the bar, but we don't know why the idiot gets through law school and passes the bar."

René Descartes' greatest fame came from proclaiming, *"Cogito, ergo sum"*–"I think, therefore I am." Sam Johnson responded with–according to a professor of mine (although I can't find a confirming reference)–"You stink, therefore you must be." I would tell Descartes that he erred, therefore he must have been. I'm not going to spend much of my life wandering through the wonders of philosophy, but when I was looking for the supposed Johnson reference, I came across *"Coito, ergo sum"*–"I fuck, therefore I am."

More simply: "What's it all about, Alfie?" Or the last words of the movie *Kids*, "Jesus Christ, what has happened?"

I find I am the happiest when I take my little bottle of Bic Wite-Out and just obliterate the philosophical quests of the ages. There is no religion that is believed by more people than disbelieved. Determinism versus free will will not be resolved before perpetual motion is achieved. For what purpose should I assign to myself the task of resolving or achieving either? I accept that I am here, and I get to love or hate, fear my emotions or embrace them, and do what I want to do about what comes at me. I can't live as happily without using everything in this book as a starter.

My character was formed in a milieu wherein I depended on love and nurture in order to survive, and my body's needs are no more or less real than those of my psyche. My life brings me the most happiness when I am kind, am responsible, ejaculate a lot, pay my bills, get enough exercise, stay healthy, love a lot, share with those in want, help those in need, and eat enough fiber.

*"There is no cure for birth and death
save to enjoy the interval."*

GEORGE SANTAYANA

END OF PART THREE

Glossary

A ass – Mr. Bumble's description of the law in *Oliver Twist*

Abasement – A lowering of respect in any sense, even the vaguest sense of frustration

Act of God – Anything not understood

Adultery – Condition, qualities, or activities acquired by growing up

Ass – A big-eared animal, or the buttocks

Asshole – Anus; part of the body, which is being insulted when George W. Bush is called one

BA – See Born Again

Bad – Whatever one doesn't like

Believers – People who form ideas based on nothing objective or scientific

Bogy – Something that functions as an imagined barrier that must be overcome

Born Again (n.) – One who is disabused of Bullshit

Born Again (v. past part) – Birthed again, this time with a mind free of Bullshit

BS – See Bullshit

Bullshit – Conditioning done to an infant predisposing the infant to blame/shame/guilt

Clarke, Arthur C. – Co-writer of screenplay *2001: A Space Odyssey*

Diamond Rule – The guide that puts the values of others in focus

Dirty Waffle – Sandy Eggo: San Diego

Donner Party – 1846 pioneers who took some bad advice and became cannibals

Doubters – People who form ideas based only on objectivity and science

E Coupon – A ticket for a ride on a top-tier attraction at Disneyland, 1959

Emotion – A state of consciousness experiencing joy, sadness, anger, fear, love, or the like

Evil – Something one really hates

Existential – Referring to what is, not what one is reacting to in one's mind

Fuck – Sexual intercourse, or an abstract syllable used for emphasis by motivational speakers

Gas – The product of a fart

Golden Rule – The guide that puts one's own values in focus

Good – What one likes

Gospel – The good news that no one needs salvation

Group A – The community of persons who like you

Group B – The riffraff of persons who don't like you

Hairsplitting – Careful differentiation beyond what is commonly achieved

Happiness – Mental health

Hives – Red, raised, intensely itchy spots usually caused by allergies; urticaria

Infancy – Condition, qualities, or activities of one who has not grown up

Infantile Omnipotence – The belief of an infant that all the universe revolves around them

Intimacy – Accepting and not manipulating one who also accepts and doesn't manipulate

Joy – The emotion of happiness caused by contentment

Kubrick, Stanley – Co-writer of screenplay and director of movie *2001: A Space Odyssey*

LAX – Los Angeles International Airport

Making Love – Rubbing against another with the expectation of emotional bonding

Masturbation – Delightful activities done with the genitals for no reason other than fun

McMartin Preschool – Manhattan Beach, CA, site of 1983 encore of Salem witch trials

Mental Masturbation – Useless activities done with the mind for no reason other than ego

Morality – A more fancy word for fantasied goodness

Myth – A legendary story which may or may not have a basis in reality

Nuremberg – World War II war crimes trials, Europe

Olduvai Gorge – Important paleoanthropological site in Tanzania

Popsicle Sticks – Polarity vehicles

Psycho-microscope – Device for the eye of the mind

Rats – An expletive which is an alternative to fuck for those, like me, who prefer not to use fuck

Rashomon – 1950 Japanese film, now considered one of the greatest films ever made

Shift of Blame – The tipping of a metaphorical balance scale to accuse another rather than self

Smudge Pots – Outdoor oil burners used to protect orange groves from frost

SOB – See Shift of Blame

Sou – From the French, a worthless coin

Sport Fucking – Rubbing against another without the expectation of emotional bonding

Symptom – A mental or physical sign that something is not as we wish

Trinity – Code name of the first detonation of a nuclear weapon

WWJD – What would Jesus do?

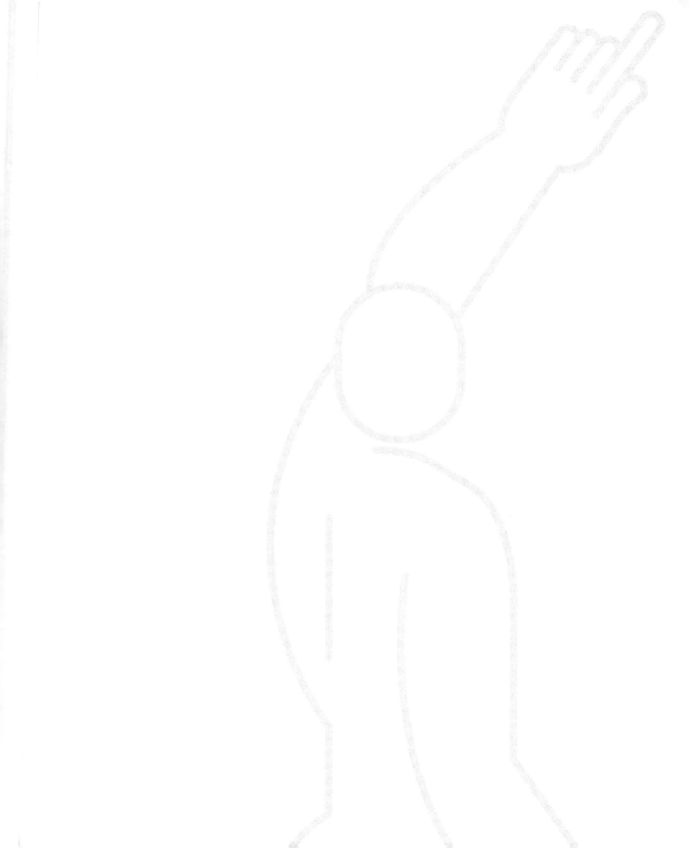

CPSIA information can be obtained
at www.ICGtesting.com
Printed in the USA
LVHW022327090122
708166LV00006B/187